RAND NATIONAL DEFENSE RESEARCH INSTITUTE

Identifying Future Disease Hot Spots

Infectious Disease Vulnerability Index

Melinda Moore, Bill Gelfeld, Adeyemi Okunogbe, Christopher Paul

T0308371

Prepared for the Office of the Secretary of Defense

For more information on this publication, visit www.rand.org/t/RR1605

Library of Congress Cataloging-in-Publication Data is available for this publication.
ISBN: 978-0-8330-9574-9

Published by the RAND Corporation, Santa Monica, Calif.
© Copyright 2016 RAND Corporation
RAND® is a registered trademark.

Cover illustration adapted from iStock/Photoraidz.

www.rand.org

Preface

Recent high-profile infectious disease outbreaks, such as those caused by the Ebola and Zika viruses, serve as a reminder of the importance of preventing, promptly detecting, and effectively limiting outbreaks, no matter where or when they emerge. This report provides an assessment of potential future disease hot spots—those countries that might be especially vulnerable to infectious disease outbreaks. This report builds on a proof of concept that RAND Corporation researchers published in March 2015. This report represents a more robust approach toward vulnerability assessment in four ways: a more comprehensive evidence base, a more robust set of factors potentially contributing to outbreak vulnerability and associated proxy measures, the use of adjustable weights for these parameters, and an examination of all countries worldwide. The assessment algorithm described in the report is inherently applicable to all outbreak-prone infectious diseases. The report describes a user-friendly tool that can help the U.S. Department of Defense, the U.S. Department of Health and Human Services and other U.S. government agencies, and international partners set priorities for technical and funding support to countries that may be most vulnerable to disease outbreaks with transnational potential.

This research was conducted within the International Security and Defense Policy Center of the RAND National Defense Research Institute, a federally funded research and development center sponsored by the Office of the Secretary of Defense, the Joint Staff, the Unified Combatant Commands, the Navy, the Marine Corps, the defense agencies, and the defense Intelligence Community.

For more information on the International Security and Defense Policy Center, see www.rand.org/nsrd/ndri/centers/isdp or contact the director (contact information is provided on the web page).

Contents

Figures and Tables

Figures

Tables

Summary

Recent high-profile outbreaks, such as those caused by the Ebola and Zika viruses, have illustrated the transnational nature of infectious diseases and the need for coordinated actions to curtail the outbreaks. Countries that are most vulnerable to such outbreaks might be higher priorities for technical and funding support. To help identify these countries, we created the Infectious Disease Vulnerability Index. This index was designed as a tool for U.S. government and international agencies to provide a clearer understanding of countries' vulnerabilities to infectious disease and thereby to help inform decisionmaking and actions about taking preemptive steps to mitigate the effects of potential widespread outbreaks.

We employed a rigorous methodology to identify the countries most vulnerable to disease outbreaks. This report builds on a proof of concept we published in the context of the Ebola outbreak (Gelfeld et al., 2015). We conducted a comprehensive review of relevant literature to identify factors influencing vulnerability to infectious disease outbreaks, which we organized into seven broad domains: demographic, health care, public health, disease dynamics, political-domestic, political-international, and economic. Using widely available data (e.g., from the World Bank, the World Health Organization, and other international organizations), we created a tool to generate an index that allows us to identify and rank potentially vulnerable countries. The tool is built to enable user-adjusted weights for individual parameters and for domains as a whole. We drew from both the rigorous literature review and our extensive experiences in epidemiology, global health, and the social sciences to create a baseline set of weights and outputs and then carried out sensitivity analyses by systematically varying the weights across all domains.

Key findings from our assessment include a heat map reflecting normed scores for all countries worldwide with regard to their vulnerability to infectious disease outbreaks (Figure S.1) and a ranked list of countries based on their vulnerability. Unsurprisingly, 22 of the 25 most-vulnerable countries are in the Africa region (within the Department of Defense's U.S. Africa Command area of responsibility); the other three are Afghanistan and Yemen (within U.S. Central Command) and Haiti (within U.S. Southern Command). Sensitivity testing first removed all weighting (i.e., all weights set to 1.0) and then systematically zeroed out (i.e., weight set to

Figure S.1
Infectious Disease Vulnerability Index World Map

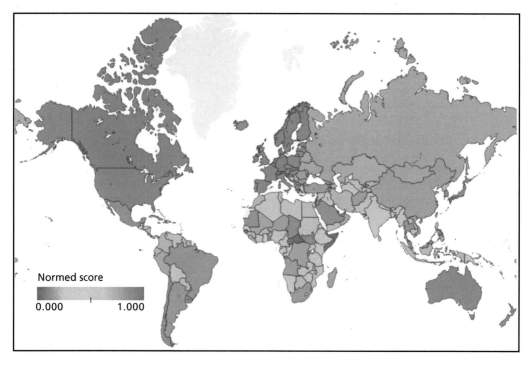

NOTE: The color shading runs from deep red (most vulnerable) to deep green (least vulnerable).
RAND *RR1605-S.1*

zero), doubled and tripled each domain weight. This testing indicated that most of the top-25 (i.e., most-vulnerable) countries remained within that range, albeit at different rankings, suggesting that the tool is highly robust to variability of parameter values from the perspective of the ranking country's vulnerability to infectious disease outbreaks. Of particular concern are conflict-affected countries, such as Somalia (ranked 1), Central African Republic (ranked 2), and South Sudan (ranked 4), all of which play host to a dangerous combination of political instability and compromised health systems.

To support our interpretation of the findings, we compared health outcomes in seven countries affected by Ebola in 2014. This comparison suggested that a high vulnerability score alone does not necessarily condemn a country to poor outcomes with regard to disease outbreaks.

We would encourage policymakers to focus on the most-vulnerable countries, with an eye toward a potential "disease belt" in the Sahel region, which emerged from the data. Of note, the vulnerability score for several countries was better than what would have been predicted on the basis of economic indicators alone. This suggests that low-income countries can overcome economic challenges and become more resilient to public health challenges.

Our aim in designing this algorithm is to provide a useful tool for U.S. federal agencies and national and international health planners worldwide to help identify and raise awareness of those countries that might be most vulnerable to infectious disease outbreaks. The algorithm can be used to guide strategic planning and programming to address vulnerabilities in health systems or other critical sectors and hone in on cases of critical geographic, demographic, or regional importance. This tool highlights the connections between economic development, political stability, and disease vulnerability. With this information in mind, the Department of Defense, the Department of Health and Human Services (e.g., through the Centers for Disease Control and Prevention), the U.S. Agency for International Development, and the international community more broadly can take targeted actions to shore up weak health systems and help countries prepare for future infectious disease outbreaks with the potential for transnational spread. Such agencies should continue or ramp up programming to strengthen public health systems (e.g., disease surveillance, laboratory testing, outbreak detection, rapid response reams for investigation and disease-control measures), as well as medical care systems (e.g., professional training and certification, clinic and hospital care). Aid organizations, such as the U.S. Agency for International Development, should also continue to promote economic development and efforts to strengthen governance. For example, better governance through democracy-promotion and anti-corruption programs may lead to less vulnerability as states improve the coordination, communication, and infrastructure systems that help to combat infectious disease transmission. Finally, exercises, including tabletop exercises, can be used to help countries better understand actions and actors, and the coordination needed among them, to best prepare systems to respond effectively to a disease threat that arises. With the multitude of disease threats that exist and the expanded opportunities for transmission in an increasingly globalized world, it is important to act now to better ensure that countries around the world, and especially the most-vulnerable countries, develop the enduring capabilities they need to effectively prevent, detect, and respond to disease threats before they get out of hand.

Acknowledgments

We would like to thank RAND's National Defense Research Institute for its generous support of this project. We would also like to thank our RAND colleagues, Seth Jones and Michael McNerney, for their leadership, insights, and inputs, and Stephanie Young of RAND and CAPT Paul Reed of the Department of Defense for their careful and thoughtful reviews of the manuscript.

CHAPTER ONE

Introduction

Recent high-profile outbreaks of Ebola, Middle East Respiratory Syndrome (MERS), pandemic influenza, and Zika, among others, have illustrated the transnational nature of infectious diseases and the need for coordinated actions to curtail them. The Global Health Security Agenda (GHSA), launched in February 2014 by the White House, along with other partner countries and organizations, aims to help countries build their capabilities to prevent, detect, and respond to infectious disease threats. GHSA does not, however, include activities to assess the relative vulnerability of countries to such threats. Which countries are most vulnerable to infectious disease outbreaks that may cross national borders and spark regional or even global spread? Such countries might be higher priorities for technical and funding support from U.S. government agencies, as well as from other partner countries and organizations.

Global health security has become a policy priority of the United States and countries around the world, enshrined explicitly in the U.S. National Security Strategy (White House, 2015), the GHSA (White House, 2014), and the U.S. National Health Security Strategy (U.S. Department of Health and Human Services [HHS], 2015). The World Health Organization's (WHO's) International Health Regulations (WHO, 2005) also fundamentally aim to enhance *global health security*, albeit without using the term explicitly. Past analyses have described the distribution of specific diseases and the overall threat of infectious diseases worldwide (see, for example, Noah and Fidas, 2000; Christian et al., 2013), but we were unable to uncover past analyses in the more than 30 studies we reviewed in the course of our literature review that systematically aimed to identify country vulnerability to infectious disease outbreaks. Given the unpredictability and potential enormity of such threats to global health security, we developed the comprehensive Infectious Disease Vulnerability Index to assess potential future disease hot spots. We created an interactive algorithm to estimate the relative vulnerability of the world's countries to infectious disease outbreaks and inform our understanding of the most potentially vulnerable countries. By *vulnerability*, we refer mainly to a country's ability to limit the spread of outbreak-prone diseases. More-vulnerable countries are less able to prevent, detect, and respond to disease spread, whereas more-resilient countries are better able to do so. While the first case (or cases) of a disease may not be entirely preventable, countries should be able to quickly detect the disease and limit its spread. The Ebola crisis in 2014–2015 illustrated both the vulnerability of certain countries and the ability of others to react quickly to overcome potential vulnerabilities and contain the disease. Most important, that crisis served as a reminder of the interconnectedness of the global community with regard to outbreak-prone infectious diseases and the importance of prevention; early detection; and timely, effective response to outbreaks, wherever and whenever they may emerge.

Assessment of potential disease hot spots complements other efforts directed toward global health security, such as direct efforts to help improve the prevention, detection, and control of transnational infectious disease threats. The assessment described here can inform prioritization for technical and funding support for such efforts, before outbreaks emerge and as soon as possible once they do emerge, thereby helping the most-vulnerable countries develop the enduring capabilities they need to prevent and control such threats.

This report is a direct follow-up to RAND's *Mitigating the Impact of Ebola in Potential Hot Zones* (Gelfeld et al., 2015), which described a proof-of-concept approach to help decisionmakers systematically assess the risk of the spread of the Ebola virus to other potentially vulnerable countries and consider actions that could be taken to mitigate the impact of Ebola in such countries. In our previous report, we recommended the further development of the algorithm to incorporate a more rigorous, quantitative methodology to systematically assess countries' vulnerability to infectious diseases. This report directly addresses that recommendation with an algorithm that is more robust in four important ways: an evidence base that is more thoroughly grounded in scholarly research and empirical studies; a more robust set of factors potentially contributing to outbreak vulnerability, along with one or more associated proxy measures for each factor; the introduction of adjustable weights for these factors and measures; and the application of the algorithm to all countries worldwide rather than just a select few.

Our aim in designing this algorithm is to provide a useful tool for U.S. federal agencies and national and international health planners worldwide to help identify and raise awareness of those countries that might be most vulnerable to infectious disease outbreaks. The algorithm can be used to guide strategic planning and programming to address health system vulnerabilities and hone in on cases of critical geographic, demographic, or regional importance. With this additional information in mind, the U.S. Department of Defense (DoD), HHS, other U.S. government agencies, and the international community more broadly can take targeted actions to shore up weak health systems and help countries prepare for future infectious disease outbreaks with the potential for transnational spread. With the multitude of disease threats that exist and the expanded opportunities for transmission in an increasingly globalized world, it is important to act now to better ensure that countries around the world, and especially the most-vulnerable countries, develop the enduring capabilities they need to effectively prevent, detect, and respond to disease threats before they get out of hand.

This report describes the Infectious Disease Vulnerability Index tool and details its potential applications as a decision-support tool for governments and international organizations. Chapter Two details the methodology behind the design of the tool. Chapter Three describes the development of the tool, its structure, and our approach to weighting the various elements. Chapter Four presents our findings from the application of the tool to all 195 countries and discusses the interpretation of the results. Chapter Five discusses potential applications of the tool for use by the United States and other governments and international organizations.

CHAPTER TWO

Methods

To better measure the key concepts of vulnerability and resilience, which we consider to be opposite sides of the same coin, we elected to use a methodology that combined rigorous literature review and expert elicitation because it has worked in similar studies and is firmly grounded in the relevant scholarly research. We first conducted an extensive literature review of the relevant scholarship on infectious disease outbreaks. Specifically, we comprehensively examined the scholarly literature that made connections between the performance of health systems and the incidence of infectious disease, through a variety of social science lenses (see the bibliography). Based on our findings, we then created a framework of factors and associated measures that followed from the central themes and conclusions identified in the relevant literature. We drew on numerous empirical studies and journal articles to identify major themes and factors pertaining to infectious diseases and country vulnerability. For each such factor (e.g., medical care workforce, corruption), we stated the thesis from the literature explaining the link between the factor and a country's vulnerability to disease outbreaks (or resilience). Based on key themes emerging from our literature review, we divided these factors into seven overarching domains: demographic, health care, public health, disease dynamics, political-domestic, political-international, and economic.

To assign a value for each factor, we matched each one with one or more proxy measures. We populated a matrix of all measures for all countries with widely available data, drawn from such sources as the World Bank and the WHO. Of note, certain data were not available for some countries. We normed the raw data for each measure to produce a numerical score between 0 (worst) and 1 (best). Also, for purposes of consistency, we arithmetically "flipped" measures for which a high score was inherently worse (e.g., infant mortality rate, corruption index).

To deal effectively with missing values, we imputed the values for missing data for a country by taking the mean value of a measure for a similar subgrouping of countries based on per capita gross domestic product (GDP) and geographic region (see Appendix B for a full listing of country subgroups). This technique divided the data into subcategories, first based on per capita income (using the five designations used by the World Bank: low income; lower middle income; upper middle income; high income, non-OECD [Organisation for Economic Co-operation and Development]; and high income, OECD) and then based on World Bank geographic region (sub-Saharan Africa, South Asia, East Asia and Pacific, Latin America and the Caribbean, the Middle East and North Africa, Europe and Central Asia, and North America). By conditioning these means on smaller bins of relevant country data generated using both per capita income and geography, we can ensure the closest matches possible and that the imputed means will therefore be as close as possible to the missing country value.

We assigned initial weights, usually between 0 and 1, to each factor and measure based on six criteria that reflect the factor's quality and credibility. The first four criteria relate to the factor itself, and the final two relate to the measure. The six criteria are (1) strength of the correlation or association between the factor and disease risk; (2) quality of the research supporting the factor; (3) face validity of the factor (does it make intuitive sense?); (4) uniqueness (the extent to which the factor is duplicative to other factors); (5) proxy value (the extent to which the measure is an effective proxy for the factor—i.e., reflecting the factor); and (6) quality of the data available for the measure. Weights for the first and second criteria emerged from findings during the literature review. Weights for the third and fourth ones were derived from our team's assessment of the factor in question. Weights for the fifth and sixth criteria are specifically related to the individual measures and are derived from the team members' evaluation according to their relevant area expertise. Where more than one measure represents a factor, the measure weights are equally distributed across the measures for the factor, to contribute to an overall factor score. We applied all of these weights to the normed raw data to calculate an indexed vulnerability score for each country and then normed that overall vulnerability score across all countries to a value between 0 and 1, with 0 indicating the country most vulnerable to infectious disease outbreaks and 1 indicating the most resilient country.

Our algorithm allows users to vary the weights based on their own assumptions, priorities, or planning requirements. To assess the overall validity of our initial weights and algorithm, we performed a number of sensitivity tests—systematically varying the weights for each domain and comparing these results with those from our initial baseline.

We recognize that there are other empirically valid ways that we might have gone about structuring this study methodologically. One such way would have been to use historical regression analysis to examine the effect on a dependent variable (infectious disease vulnerability) of a host of independent variables to test their effects on the outcome in question. While empirically rigorous, this methodology has challenges of its own given that historical regression analysis is not unproblematic. There are counterfactual concerns in addition to establishing the necessary distinction between vulnerability (the potential effects and extent of a disease outbreak should it occur) and risk (the confluence of the likelihood of, the vulnerability to, and the consequences of a disease outbreak) in this context. Furthermore, given the effort required and the challenges faced because of missing data in assembling recent and contemporary data for all countries, assembling global historical data for any significant period would have been nontrivial.

CHAPTER THREE

Developing a Framework to Assess Vulnerability

Throughout the course of our literature review and research, we found that the most-relevant concepts and associated measures fell into seven common domains within the four broader thematic categories of demographic, health, political, and economic factors. The seven domains are demographic, health care, public health, disease dynamics, political-domestic, political-international, and economic. Factors and associated measures within these seven domains provide the framework for our quantitative analysis.

Framework Foundation: Seven Domains and Associated Factors

The sections that follow describe the factors within each domain, and Figure 3.1 provides an overall summary. In the course of our initial literature review, we found well-regarded academic studies linking every factor to vulnerability to infectious diseases. We derived the domains by organizing the factors by theme. In total, we used approximately three dozen different studies to establish these connections to verify our hypotheses and lay the intellectual foundation for the tool. Our list of data sources and bibliography (at the end of this report) are both organized by domain.

Demographic Factors
Several demographic factors influence the degree of vulnerability of a country to infectious disease outbreaks. The relevant literature emphasizes the role of such factors as population density, growth and mobility, and the degree of urbanization. States with densely packed, fast-growing urban areas and high population mobility across borders are more vulnerable to the spread of contagious diseases. The level of education or literacy can also play a helpful role in mitigating the spread and effects of infectious diseases by enhancing the adoption of health behaviors or practices that reduce disease transmission.

Figure 3.1
Domains and Factors Associated with Disease Outbreak Vulnerability

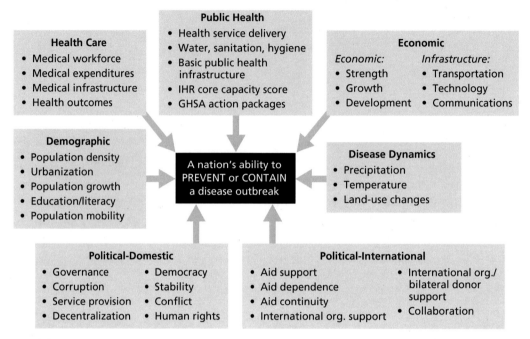

Health Care Factors

The strength and quality of a nation's health care system have an obvious and direct bearing on resiliency to infectious disease outbreaks. This is supported by a large body of published evidence. From our extensive literature review, we included key factors that indicate the strength of national health systems and selected proxy measures to represent them. Factors include the size of the medical care workforce (doctors and nurses), health care expenditures, and health care infrastructure (number of different types of health care facilities). Based on the relevant research, we also included a measure—infant mortality rate—as an indicator of the health status of a country.

Public Health Factors

Strong public health systems are needed to ensure that a country can prevent, promptly detect, and effectively respond to infectious disease outbreaks. The ability of a government to deliver basic health services (such as vaccinations) and the proportion of the population with access to clean water and improved sanitation facilities reflect how well communities can prevent or respond to disease threats. The extent to which a country has developed its core public health capacities in accordance with the WHO's International Health Regulations (IHR) or the degree of direct engagement in GHSA should, in principle, also serve as important indicators of the adequacy of the country's public health system and, hence, its resilience against disease outbreaks.

Disease Dynamics Factors

Climate-related and ecological factors can also influence a country's vulnerability to disease outbreaks. Patterns of precipitation and temperature can directly affect disease transmission through impacts on the replication and movement (and perhaps evolution) of disease microbes and vectors giving rise to water- or vector-borne diseases, such as cholera, malaria, dengue, and West Nile virus. Furthermore, evidence suggests that increases in anthropogenic activities—such as changes in the national patterns of land use, including the extent of agricultural activities and deforestation—are associated with the likelihood of emergence of zoonotic infectious diseases. This process happens either by increasing proximity to conditions or, often, by changing the conditions that favor an increased population of the microbe or its natural host. Accordingly, we have accounted for these factors in our model.

Political-Domestic Factors

Domestic political factors can also affect the ability of a government to prepare for and respond to infectious disease outbreaks and thus will have a significant bearing on its vulnerability to such threats. Backed by several academic studies, we have posited that governance (measured by three different World Bank governance indicators) has a positive effect on resiliency, while corruption has a deleterious one. Stable governments without conflicts within their borders are also likely to be more resilient in this regard, as are governments that are perceived as providing quality services to their citizens. Furthermore, greater levels of democracy and political decentralization, along with respect for human rights, are associated with a state's ability to defend itself against disease threats. Greater levels of democracy within a country and empowerment of local government often yield more-capable organization and response at the city, state, or province level. Successful decentralization creates several levels of contingency response throughout a country that can set up mechanisms to respond to a disease outbreak. Civil society organizations, generally more vibrant and participative in a democracy, can also help prepare for and respond to disease outbreaks. Furthermore, respect for human rights means that citizens feel more empowered to provide feedback regarding prevention and response efforts so that mechanisms in place to prevent the spread of diseases are more fully vetted by citizen interest groups.

Political-International Factors

Along with domestic considerations, international political factors affect a country's resilience to infectious disease outbreaks. The consistent support of both bilateral donors and international organizations can help strengthen a country's health system and provide critical funding, expertise, and personnel in preparing for and responding to health crises. The response of the WHO; the U.S. Centers for Disease Control and Prevention (CDC); and various nongovernmental organizations (NGOs), such as Médecins Sans Frontières (Doctors Without Borders), among others, proved crucial in containing the Ebola crisis in West Africa. While aid can certainly help mitigate the effects of infectious diseases, studies have shown that aid can also create dangerous dependencies, a fact that we have reflected in our algorithm.

Economic Factors

The size and scope of a country's economy often dictates the amount and quality of resources it has to prepare for and respond to the threats posed by infectious diseases. As a result, we incorporated certain measures of economic strength and development into our model, including GDP per capita, economic growth rates, the Human Development Index (from the United Nations Development Programme), and national poverty ratios. Academic research into infectious diseases also pointed to the importance of communications and transportation infrastructure and the technological sophistication of a society; as result, we have included these factors and associated measures into our model.

Assembling the Framework and Assigning Weights

Weights acted as multipliers in calculating the overall vulnerability score. Weighting values were assigned separately for each parameter and also for a domain as a whole. Tables 3.1–3.7 summarize the factors, hypotheses, measures, and initial assigned weights for the seven domains. We drew from both our rigorous literature review and our collective expertise and experiences in the fields of epidemiology, health, and social science in assigning these initial weights. We adopted a convention of assigning weights mostly in the range of 0 to 1.0 for each factor and measure, mostly in increments of 0.25 (e.g., 0.25, 0.50, 0.75) and preferably not all clustering around 1.0. A weight of 0 for any of the six criteria effectively eliminates the factor from the calculations. We did not assign a zero weight to any parameter in our baseline scenario. As the perceived value of each factor or measure increased, we increased the numerical value assigned to the respective weights from 0 and approached 1.0 (or beyond, if weights greater than 1.0 were assigned). We considered four factors to be of particular importance and assigned baseline weights greater than 1.0 for the strength of correlation parameter (ρ): We assigned a weight of 2.0 for a composite IHR core capacity score, governance, and government stability and a weight of 1.5 to a factor reflecting economic strength. Because we deemed these to be the most-influential factors in terms of their significant, direct impact on disease vulnerability, we assigned them weights greater than 1.0. The significance of these specific factors was determined through the confluence of their importance in both the relevant literature and our professional judgment.

We assigned weights for six parameters related to each factor. Strength of correlation (ρ) is intended to be the equivalent of a regression coefficient, had the parameter been derived based on regression; ρ denotes the strength of correlation between the factor and the outcome as identified in existing research. Quality of research (Q_r) captures our holistic assessment of the strength of evidence in support of the contribution of the factor as marshaled in the existing research. Where multiple highly rigorous studies inform the factor, this weight is (or approaches) 1.0; where fewer studies with thinner empirical foundation inform the factor, weights are lower. No factor has a quality-of-research assessment lower than 0.5, because any factor with such a slim foundation was entirely eliminated from consideration. Face validity (F) captures our assessment of the face validity of the identified correlation. A face validity value below 1 indicates that we are skeptical about the strength of correlation proposed in the informing literature (that is, we believe that the factor is important but that it is not as strongly correlated as existing research suggests) or that we can imagine alternative mechanisms that diminish our confidence in the importance of the factor. Uniqueness (R) denotes the extent to which the factor is redundant with other factors. While each factor is distinct, they are not necessarily discrete. We included uniqueness to reduce the overall weight where we have included several similar and related factors. Proxy value (X) denotes our assessment of the extent to which the measure used is a good representative of the factor. A proxy value weight of 1.0 indicates that the measure is a perfect match for the factor, while lower weights indicate that the best measure we were able to find for the factor is less than ideal. The quality of data weight (Q_d) is similar, being 1.0 where the data used to represent the factor are of the highest quality and being lower where the data are beset by measurement error, low currency (that is, are somewhat out-of-date), or extensive missing information.

These six weights combine with the data representing each factor for each country in the following way. First, the raw data for a measure of a factor are normed across all countries over the range 0 to 1.0. Then, the normed measure for each country is multiplied by all six weights for the factor. Finally, the weighted measures are normed again across all countries to produce a factor score for each country ranging between 0 and 1.0, where the worst country in the data scores 0 for the factor and the best country scores 1.0. To generate scores for domains, all factor scores within a domain are summed for each country and then normed again across countries. To generate overall scores for each country, all factors across all domains are summed by country and then normed across countries. So, at each level (individual factor, domain, or overall), each score ranges between 0 and 1.0, with the worst country on that factor, domain, or overall scoring 0 and the best country scoring 1.0.

The results presented here reflect the strength of correlations in publications, the quality of the data available, and judgments of the authors. The tool was constructed to enable users to adjust weights, as we did with our initial weightings and the subsequent sensitivity testing (described in Chapter Four). Because the method adopted for imputing missing values rendered the tool less user-friendly, the tool is not published online but is available by request from the authors. Different users may have different priorities and hence may wish to assign significantly different weights. One can imagine, for example, that security sector planners (e.g., DoD) might assign higher weights to security-related parameters, whereas health sector planners (e.g., HHS, the U.S. Agency for International Development [USAID]) might assign higher weights to health-related parameters, and yet others might consider economic factors to be most important and wish to adjust the assigned weights accordingly.

Table 3.1
Demographic Factors, Hypotheses, Measures, and Weights

Label	Factor	Hypothesis	Measure	Weights					
				ρ	Q_r	F	R	X	Q_d
DG-1	Population density	A country with higher population density is more susceptible to the spread of emerging infectious diseases via overcrowding	Persons per square km (high = bad; flip measure value)	0.75	1.00	0.75	0.25	1.00	0.90
DG-2	Urbanization (interaction with water, sanitation, hygiene)	A country with densely populated urban areas is more susceptible to the spread of infectious diseases via overcrowding and direct or indirect contact with numerous persons	Percentage of persons living in urban areas (high = bad; flip measure value)	0.75	0.90	0.75	0.25	1.00	0.90
DG-3	Human population growth	A country with higher growth in population is more susceptible to the spread of emerging infectious diseases via overcrowding	Annual population growth rate (average annual percentage change in population) (high = bad; flip measure value)	0.50	0.90	0.50	0.25	1.00	0.90
DG-4	Education/ literacy	A country with high rates of literacy and education is less susceptible to the spread of emerging diseases via risky behaviors that may increase exposure	Adult literacy rate (high = good)	0.75	0.90	1.00	1.00	1.00	0.90
			Adult female literacy rate (high = good)	0.75	0.90	1.00	1.00	1.00	0.90
DG-5	Population mobility	A country with high migration and mobility of peoples is more susceptible to the spread of infectious diseases	Net migration rate (average annual number of migrants per 1,000 people) (high = bad; flip measure value)	0.50	0.50	0.75	1.00	0.75	0.90

NOTES: Factor weights are ρ = strength of correlation; Q_r = quality of research; F = face validity; R = redundancy (uniqueness). Measure weights are X = proxy value; Q_d = quality of data.

Table 3.2
Health Care Factors, Hypotheses, Measures, and Weights

Label	Factor	Hypothesis	Measure	ρ	Q_r	F	R	X	Q_d
						Weights			
HC-1	Medical care workforce	A country with more health care providers is better able to limit infectious disease outbreaks	Number of physicians per 1,000 population (high = good)	0.90	0.50	0.75	1.00	1.00	0.65
			Number of nurses and midwives per 1,000 population (high = good)	0.90	0.50	0.75	1.00	1.00	0.65
HC-2	Medical care expenditures	A country with greater spending on health (specifically, health care) is better able to limit infectious disease outbreaks	Percentage of GDP spent on health (high = good)	0.50	0.90	0.50	0.33	1.00	0.90
			Health expenditure per capita (high = good)	0.50	0.90	0.50	0.33	1.00	0.90
HC-3	Medical care infrastructure	A country with a better medical infrastructure is better able to respond to limit infectious disease outbreaks	Hospital beds per 1,000 population (high = good)	0.50	0.70	0.75	0.33	1.00	0.90
			Health posts per 100,000 population (high = good)	0.50	0.70	0.75	0.33	1.00	0.90
			Health centers per 100,000 population (high = good)	0.50	0.70	0.75	0.33	1.00	0.90
			Hospitals per 100,000 population (high = good)	0.50	0.70	0.75	0.33	1.00	0.90
HC-4	Health status/ outcomes	A country with worse health status, with infant mortality rate as a proxy, reflects less ability to deliver services and in turn is less able to respond effectively to prevent or limit infectious disease outbreaks	Infant mortality rate (number of deaths in <12 months per 1,000 live births) (high = bad; flip measure value)	0.75	0.90	1.00	1.00	1.00	0.90

NOTES: Factor weights are ρ = strength of correlation; Q_r = quality of research; F = face validity; R = redundancy (uniqueness). Measure weights are X = proxy value; Q_d = quality of data.

Table 3.3
Public Health Factors, Hypotheses, Measures, and Weights

Label	Factor	Hypothesis	Measure	Weights					
				ρ	Q_r	F	R	X	Q_d
PH-1	Health service delivery	A country that is better able to deliver basic primary care services is also better able to respond to limit the spread of infectious disease outbreaks	Percentage coverage with third dose of DTP vaccine (high = good)	0.90	0.50	1.00	0.33	1.00	0.90
			Percentage coverage with first dose of measles vaccine (high = good)	0.90	0.50	1.00	0.33	1.00	0.90
PH-2	Water, sanitation, and hygiene infrastructure	A country with more widespread availability of potable water, sanitary conditions, and proper hygiene is better protected against the transmission of some infectious diseases—e.g., cholera	Population using improved drinking-water sources (%) (high = good)	1.00	0.90	1.00	1.00	1.00	0.90
			Population using improved sanitation facilities (%) (high = good)	1.00	0.90	1.00	1.00	1.00	0.90
PH-3	Basic public health infrastructure	A country with a strong public health infrastructure—e.g., having a national public health institute—is better able to prevent and respond effectively to limit infectious disease outbreaks	Country is member of the International Association of National Public Health Institutes (binary; 1 = yes [good])	0.50	0.75	1.00	1.00	0.75	0.90
PH-4	Composite IHR core capacity score	A country with stronger IHR core capacities is better able to prevent and respond effectively to limit infectious disease outbreaks	Arithmetic average of score across all IHR scores (high = good)	2.00	0.90	1.00	1.00	1.00	0.90
PH-5	GHSA action packages	A country that is committed to lead or contribute to a GHSA action package will be better able to contain infectious disease outbreaks	Country leading or contributing to >1 GHSA action package (binary; 1 = yes [good])	0.25	0.90	0.75	1.00	0.75	0.90

NOTES: Factor weights are ρ = strength of correlation; Q_r = quality of research; F = face validity; R = redundancy (uniqueness). Measure weights are X = proxy value; Q_d = quality of data. DTP = diphtheria-tetanus-pertussis.

Table 3.4
Disease Dynamics Factors, Hypotheses, Measures, and Weights

Label	Factor	Hypothesis	Measure	Weights					
				ρ	Q_r	F	R	X	Q_d
Environmental factor									
DD-1	Precipitation/ rainfall	A country with greater precipitation can have greater transmission of water- and vector-borne diseases because of the effects of precipitation on the replication and movement (and perhaps evolution) of disease microbes and vectors	Average rainfall per year (mm) (high = bad; flip measure value)	0.25	0.70	0.75	1.00	0.75	0.90
DD-2	Temperature	A country with higher temperatures can have greater transmission of water- and vector-borne diseases because of the effects of temperature on the replication and movement (and perhaps evolution) of disease microbes and vectors	Annual average temperature (high = bad; flip measure value)	0.25	0.70	0.75	1.00	0.75	0.75
Ecological factor									
DD-3	Changes in land use	Increasing anthropogenic activities is associated with increased susceptibility to and likelihood of emergence of zoonotic infectious diseases—either by increasing proximity or, often, by changing conditions that favor an increased population of the microbe or its natural host	Agricultural land (%) (high = bad; flip measure value)	0.50	0.90	0.75	1.00	1.00	0.90
			Forest area (%) (high = bad; flip measure value)	0.50	0.90	0.75	1.00	1.00	0.90
			Global deforestation rates (%) (high = bad; flip measure value)	0.50	0.90	0.75	1.00	1.00	0.90

NOTES: Factor weights are ρ = strength of correlation; Q_r = quality of research; F = face validity; R = redundancy (uniqueness). Measure weights are X = proxy value; Q_d = quality of data.

Table 3.5
Political-Domestic Factors, Hypotheses, Measures, and Weights

Label	Factor	Hypothesis	Measure	Weights					
				ρ	Q_r	F	R	X	Q_d
P-D-1	Governance	A country with a competent and strong government is better able to contend with an infectious disease outbreak	Worldwide Governance Indicators Government Effectiveness Index (high = good)	2.00	0.70	1.00	1.00	1.00	0.90
			Worldwide Governance Indicators Regulatory Quality Index (high = good)	2.00	0.70	1.00	1.00	0.50	0.75
			Worldwide Governance Indicators Rule of Law Index (high = good)	2.00	0.70	1.00	1.00	0.75	0.90
P-D-2	Corruption	A country with greater corruption has worse health outcomes and greater vulnerability to infectious disease outbreaks	Transparency International Corruption Perceptions Index (high = good)	0.75	1.00	0.75	0.50	1.00	0.90
P-D-3	Service provision	A country with greater stability and better quality of services has fewer barriers (geographical, financial, personnel, and access) to health care for marginalized populations	United Nations Development Programme Human Development Report Health Systems Survey (high = good)	0.75	0.90	0.75	0.50	0.50	0.65
P-D-4	Decentral-ization	Various dynamics of decentralization (fiscal, political) are linked with positive health outcomes	World Bank decentralization index (high = good)	0.75	0.70	0.50	1.00	1.00	0.90
P-D-5	Democracy	A country with a more democratic and legitimate government is better able to contend with an infectious disease outbreak	Polity IV Project Democracy Index (high = good)	0.50	0.90	0.75	1.00	1.00	0.75
P-D-6	Government stability	State fragility increases vulnerability to infectious disease outbreaks, while infectious disease outbreaks can exacerbate existing state weaknesses	Fund for Peace Fragile States Index (high = bad; flip measure value)	2.00	0.70	1.00	0.50	1.00	0.90

Table 3.5—Continued

Label	Factor	Hypothesis	Measure	ρ	Q_r	Weights F	R	X	Q_d
P-D-7	Presence of conflict	Political stability—absence of conflict and state fragility—is associated with better ability to deliver health care and better health outcomes	Worldwide Governance Indicators Political Stability and Absence of Violence Index (World Bank) (high = good)	0.90	0.70	1.00	0.50	0.75	0.75
P-D-8	Human rights	A worse human rights record is linked with worse health performance	Amnesty International Political Terror Scale (high = bad; flip measure value)	0.50	0.58	0.50	1.00	0.50	0.25
			U.S. Department of State via Amnesty International Political Terror Scale (high = bad; flip measure value)	0.50	0.58	0.50	1.00	0.50	0.25

NOTES: Factor weights are ρ = strength of correlation; Q_r = quality of research; F = face validity; R = redundancy (uniqueness). Measure weights are X = proxy value; Q_d = quality of data.

Table 3.6
Political-International Factors, Hypotheses, Measures, and Weights

Label	Factor	Hypothesis	Measure	Weights					
				ρ	Q_r	F	R	X	Q_d
Successful cooperation with foreign partners									
P-I-1	Aid support	States receiving more donor aid are better able to ensure health system functionality	World Bank Net Official Development Assistance per capita (high = good)	0.50	0.50	0.75	0.33	0.75	0.75
P-I-2	Aid dependence	Countries with a high proportion of donor aid are less able to deal with health emergencies on their own and therefore are more vulnerable to infectious disease outbreak	World Bank Net Official Development Assistance received (% gross national income) (high = bad; flip measure value)	0.75	0.50	0.75	0.33	1.00	0.75
P-I-3	Aid continuity	Consistent, predictable funding support can promote better infectious disease control through stronger health systems	Lagged correlation between foreign aid and foreign direct investment (high = good)	0.50	0.50	0.75	0.33	0.75	0.50
International cooperation and collaboration									
P-I-4	International organization support	Greater involvement, funding, and assistance by intergovernmental or bilateral partners will lead to more-effective detection and control of infectious disease outbreak	United Nations Development Programme recipient funding by country per capita (high = good)	0.75	0.50	0.75	0.50	0.25	0.25
P-I-5	International organization/ bilateral support for health	International organization and bilateral support to developing countries should lead to health sector strengthening and better resiliency against and response to infectious disease outbreaks	Development assistance for health by country 2011 (high = good)	0.50	0.50	0.75	0.50	0.75	0.75
			Development assistance for health per capita (high = good)	0.50	0.50	0.75	0.50	0.75	0.75
P-I-6	Collaboration	Collaboration across governments, donors, and NGOs in program design and implementation is associated with better health systems and infectious disease control	Involvement with multilateral institutions (Jane's) (high = good)	0.75	0.50	0.75	1.0	0.50	0.50

NOTES: Factor weights are ρ = strength of correlation; Q_r = quality of research; F = face validity; R = redundancy (uniqueness). Measure weights are X = proxy value; Q_d = quality of data.

Table 3.7
Economic Factors, Hypotheses, Measures, and Weights

Label	Factor	Hypothesis	Measure	Weights ρ	Q_r	F	R	X	Q_d
Strong economy and strong economic growth									
EC-1	Economic strength	A strong economy is associated with better health outcomes (lower infant mortality and longer life expectancy) in all countries	GDP per capita (high = good)	1.50	0.90	1.00	0.50	0.75	0.75
EC-2	Economic growth	Greater economic growth has led to significant gains in control of infectious disease outbreaks (tuberculosis, polio) even in countries with weak institutional environments (Democratic Republic of the Congo [DRC], Myanmar, Haiti); the gains from economic growth flow directly into health gains, up to a certain threshold of development	GDP per capita growth rate (2010–2014) (high = good)	0.50	0.50	0.75	1.00	1.00	0.75
EC-3	Economic development	Countries with stronger economic development have greater access to diagnostic resources, making these countries more able to detect and respond to infectious disease outbreaks	United Nations Development Programme Human Development Index (high = good)	0.75	0.70	0.90	0.50	0.75	0.75
		Greater economic development has led to better efforts to control infectious disease as a result of more and higher-quality resources with which to combat the spread of infectious disease	Poverty headcount ratio under $1.25 per day (high = bad; flip measure value)	0.75	0.90	0.90	0.50	0.75	0.75

Table 3.7—Continued

Label	Factor	Hypothesis	Measure	Weights					
				ρ	Q_r	F	R	X	Q_d
Infrastructure and technology									
EC-4	Partner-nation transportation infrastructure	Good transportation infrastructure makes it easier to deliver needed medical supplies to a country and to distribute them throughout the country	World Bank Logistics Performance Index (high = good)	0.50	0.50	0.75	1.00	0.50	0.65
			Percentage of paved roads (of total) (high = good)					0.50	0.50
EC-5	Technological sophistication	Greater technological penetration and sophistication are associated with better infectious disease control	World Bank Knowledge Economy Index (high = good)	0.75	0.90	0.75	1.00	0.75	0.65
EC-6	Partner-nation communications infrastructure	Good communications infrastructure makes it easier to deliver information about infectious disease and control measures to the population and outlying authorities	Televisions per 1,000 people (high = good)	0.50	0.50	0.75	1.00	0.25	0.50
			Cell phone subscriptions per 100 people (high = good)					0.50	0.65
			Internet users per 100 people (high = good)					0.25	0.65

NOTES: Factor weights are ρ = strength of correlation; Q_r = quality of research; F = face validity; R = redundancy (uniqueness). Measure weights are X = proxy value; Q_d = quality of data.

CHAPTER FOUR

Results

The indexed scores—the overall score and domain-specific scores—for all countries are presented as normed values between 0 and 1.0 and are listed in ranked order in Appendix A. The global distribution of vulnerability can be seen visually in Figure 4.1. In this chapter, we first present initial results and observations about the Infectious Disease Vulnerability Index scores and then present the results of our sensitivity analysis. We then discuss the implications of our findings and use the Ebola and Zika outbreaks as examples to illustrate these results.

Initial Results

To determine vulnerability profiles, it is instructive to look at the most-vulnerable and least-vulnerable countries, as indicated by the Infectious Disease Vulnerability Index, and evaluate each list for commonalities and trends. We first present the 25 most-vulnerable countries according to our algorithm and then present, by way of contrast, the 25 least-vulnerable countries.

Most-Vulnerable Countries

Examining the 25 most-vulnerable countries (Table 4.1) reveals few surprises, with 22 of the 25 countries located in sub-Saharan Africa (covered by U.S. Africa Command [AFRICOM]). The other three countries—Haiti, Afghanistan, and Yemen—have similar profiles to the high-vulnerability African countries in terms of poor access to resources, poor governance, and weak health systems. The tables here and in Appendix A present the countries in rank order, from most to least vulnerable. Across the 195 countries, the color shading of overall normed scores runs from deep red (most vulnerable) through orange and yellow to light and deeper green (least vulnerable). The 25 most-vulnerable countries have normed scores ranging from 0 (normed minimum value, for Somalia) to 0.26 (Mozambique), shaded from deep red to light orange. The 25 least-vulnerable countries have normed scores ranging from 0.82 (Italy) to 1.0 (normed maximum value, for Norway).

Figure 4.1
Infectious Disease Vulnerability Index World Map

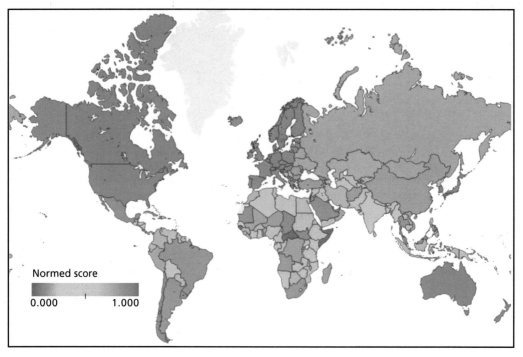

Several notable trends emerge from the full results of our model (found in Appendix A)—including overall index scores and domain-specific scores across all 195 countries—that can inform our understanding and possible responses. The first and most evident trend is the presence of conflict or recent conflict among more-vulnerable countries. Seven of the ten most-vulnerable countries are in current conflict zones (Somalia, Central African Republic, South Sudan, Afghanistan) or have had a history of recent conflict (Angola, Madagascar, Chad). Certainly, conflict undermines the strength of a country's health system and often reflects weak, divided, or even failed government. Because resources are destroyed in conflict and trained professionals are incentivized to leave, conflict further exacerbates existing problem areas, creating potential infectious disease hot spots.

Another concerning trend, which is already somewhat apparent in Figure 4.1 but shown more clearly in Figure 4.2, is geographic in nature: 24 of the 30 most-vulnerable countries form a solid, near-contiguous belt from the edge of West Africa in Mauritania, the Gambia, and Guinea through the Sahel countries of Mali, Niger, Chad, and Sudan to the Horn of Africa in Somalia—a disease hot spot belt.

Were a communicable disease to emerge within this chain of countries, it could easily spread across borders in all directions, abetted by high overall vulnerability and

Table 4.1
25 Most-Vulnerable Countries

Rank	Combatant Command	Country or Territory	Normed Score
1	AFRICOM	Somalia	0.000000
2	AFRICOM	Central African Republic	0.000061
3	AFRICOM	Chad	0.098450
4	AFRICOM	South Sudan	0.100836
5	AFRICOM	Mauritania	0.107294
6	AFRICOM	Angola	0.148414
7	SOUTHCOM	Haiti	0.149471
8	CENTCOM	Afghanistan	0.157034
9	AFRICOM	Niger	0.166531
10	AFRICOM	Madagascar	0.170787
11	AFRICOM	Democratic Republic of the Congo	0.181762
12	AFRICOM	Mali	0.184254
13	AFRICOM	Guinea-Bissau	0.187841
14	AFRICOM	Benin	0.206682
15	AFRICOM	The Gambia	0.207809
16	AFRICOM	Liberia	0.213114
17	AFRICOM	Guinea	0.213225
18	AFRICOM	São Tomé and Príncipe	0.223256
19	AFRICOM	Sierra Leone	0.223397
20	AFRICOM	Burkina Faso	0.231504
21	AFRICOM	Comoros	0.238068
22	CENTCOM	Yemen	0.250277
23	AFRICOM	Eritrea	0.252978
24	AFRICOM	Togo	0.259396
25	AFRICOM	Mozambique	0.262501

NOTES: The color shading runs from deep red (most vulnerable) to deeper green (least vulnerable). SOUTHCOM = U.S. Southern Command; CENTCOM = U.S. Central Command.

Figure 4.2
Infectious Disease Hot Spot Belt

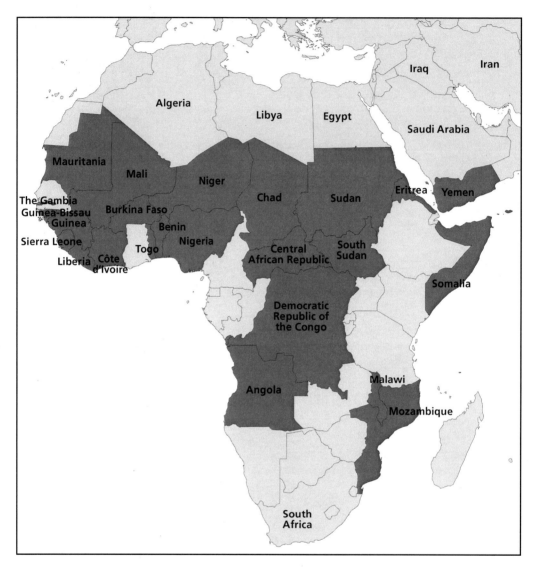

a string of weak national health systems along the way. Disease could also easily spread to the south of Africa through the vulnerable border states of DRC and Angola and to the greater Middle East from South Sudan, Eritrea, or Somalia through the gateway of Yemen. Though we have seen modern diseases rapidly transmitted all over the world through interconnected travel, it is these vulnerable states with porous borders and weak or conflict-affected neighbors that face the greatest risks and potential health challenges. As we have already witnessed with Ebola, it would not be long before these developing-world health problems appeared on the doorstep of the developed world. Solutions could be far more quickly and cost-effectively implemented in a preemptive fashion than a purely reactive one.

Least-Vulnerable Countries

Not surprisingly, the 25 least-vulnerable countries (i.e., those ranked numbers 171–195 among the 195 countries examined; see Table 4.2) are all highly developed nations in Europe, North America, and Asia-Pacific with robust democracies, economies, and health systems. The normed scores for these countries range from 0.82 (Italy) to 1.0 (Norway), and they are all shaded dark green in the red-orange-yellow-green spectrum. The six least-vulnerable countries (i.e., ranks 190 to 195) include all four Scandinavian countries, which are at the top of many composite indicators, such as the Human Development Index, and Germany and Canada; these are followed by Japan (189) and the United States (188). In comparing the 25 least-vulnerable countries against the next 25 and those progressively more vulnerable, the 25 least-vulnerable countries tend to have larger medical workforces and medical expenditures; better health indicators; less corrupt and more-stable (usually democratic) governments; better human rights; and stronger economic development, transportation infrastructure, and technological sophistication.

Results from the Sensitivity Analysis

Notwithstanding our extensive literature review and vetting of baseline weights through multiple rounds of analysis and discussion, we realize that there remains room for continued discussion in this area. To further validate our results, we systematically adjusted the domain weights to assess the nature and degree of the changes in our results. First, to test the effect of any weighting of parameters, we assigned a value of 1.0 to every parameter weight—effectively eliminating the subjective weighting scheme—to examine the effect on the country vulnerability rankings. Then, to assess changes in the relative weight of the different domains and compare those results with our baseline scenario, we systematically doubled, tripled, and zeroed out each domain weight, leaving all parameter weights at baseline values and all other domains weighted at a value of 1.0. The results of all these sensitivity tests are presented in Table 4.3.

As shown in Table 4.3, the reweighting of all parameter values to 1.0 (i.e., functionally eliminating weighting) resulted in four countries rising into the top 25 most vulnerable: Democratic People's Republic of Korea (North Korea), which rose from 46 to 3, the Republic of the Congo (Congo-Brazzaville), which rose from just outside the top 25, at 26, to 15; Sudan, which rose from 30 to 21; and Côte d'Ivoire, which rose from 28 to 24. The four countries that fell out of the top 25 most vulnerable were São Tomé and Príncipe (18 to 41), Sierra Leone (19 to 27), Burkina Faso (20 to

Table 4.2
25 Least-Vulnerable Countries

Rank	Combatant Command	Country or Territory	Normed Score
171	EUCOM	Italy	0.821690
172	EUCOM	Czech Republic	0.847175
173	EUCOM	France	0.855407
174	EUCOM	Belgium	0.870933
175	EUCOM	Austria	0.874243
176	EUCOM	Spain	0.875475
177	EUCOM	Luxembourg	0.875694
178	PACOM	Singapore	0.878289
179	PACOM	Republic of Korea (South Korea)	0.879402
180	EUCOM	Portugal	0.888782
181	EUCOM	United Kingdom	0.897495
182	EUCOM	Ireland	0.906320
183	EUCOM	Iceland	0.908112
184	PACOM	Australia	0.912517
185	EUCOM	Switzerland	0.915839
186	PACOM	New Zealand	0.916279
187	EUCOM	Netherlands	0.918935
188	NORTHCOM	United States	0.924939
189	PACOM	Japan	0.926410
190	EUCOM	Denmark	0.953641
191	EUCOM	Sweden	0.955625
192	EUCOM	Germany	0.966890
193	EUCOM	Finland	0.968274
194	NORTHCOM	Canada	0.973400
195	EUCOM	Norway	1.000000

NOTES: The color shading runs from deep red (most vulnerable) to deeper green (least vulnerable). EUCOM = U.S. European Command; NORTHCOM = U.S. Northern Command; PACOM = U.S. Pacific Command.

Table 4.3
Results of Sensitivity Testing: Adjusting Domain Weights

Baseline Rank	Country or Territory	Unweighted (all weights = 1)	Demographic			Health Care			Public Health			Disease Dynamics			Political - Domestic			Political - International			Economic		
			Double	Triple	Zero	Double	Triple	Zero	Double	Triple	Zero	Double	Triple	Zero	Double	Triple	Zero	Double	Triple	Zero	Double	Triple	Zero
1	Somalia	5	2	2	1	2	2	1	1	1	2	2	2	1	1	1	2	1	1	2	2	2	1
2	Central African Republic	1	1	1	2	1	1	2	2	2	1	1	1	2	2	2	1	2	2	1	1	1	2
3	Chad	6	4	4	4	3	3	5	4	5	3	4	4	3	4	4	4	3	3	3	3	3	5
4	South Sudan	2	3	3	5	4	6	3	5	6	4	3	3	4	3	3	6	4	4	4	4	4	3
5	Mauritania	12	5	6	3	5	5	4	3	3	16	5	5	5	5	7	3	5	5	5	5	7	4
6	Angola	17	9	12	6	6	4	10	7	7	11	7	8	6	8	9	9	6	6	7	8	9	6
7	Haiti	8	8	8	7	8	11	6	8	9	8	6	6	8	7	6	11	7	7	6	6	6	7
8	Afghanistan	16	7	7	9	7	8	8	13	17	5	9	12	7	6	5	16	8	8	8	7	5	9
9	Niger	14	6	5	13	10	12	9	9	10	15	10	10	9	11	15	7	10	10	9	10	10	8
10	Madagascar	9	12	19	8	13	16	7	6	4	35	8	7	10	14	19	5	9	9	10	9	8	11
11	Democratic Republic of the Congo	4	15	17	10	9	7	15	17	20	6	11	9	12	9	8	19	11	11	11	11	11	12
12	Mali	13	10	9	12	11	9	14	11	12	12	13	13	11	12	16	10	12	13	12	13	13	10
13	Guinea-Bissau	20	13	13	11	12	13	11	14	16	9	12	11	13	10	11	14	13	12	13	12	12	13

Rank After Adjusting Weight as Indicated

Table 4.3—Continued

Baseline Rank	Country or Territory	Unweighted (all weights = 1)	Demographic			Health Care			Public Health			Disease Dynamics			Political - Domestic			Political - International			Economic		
			Double	Triple	Zero	Double	Triple	Zero	Double	Triple	Zero	Double	Triple	Zero	Double	Triple	Zero	Double	Triple	Zero	Double	Triple	Zero
14	Benin	18	11	11	18	15	14	17	12	11	26	14	15	16	25	30	8	15	16	14	16	17	14
15	The Gambia	11	16	15	16	18	19	13	15	14	19	16	18	14	17	17	13	14	15	15	15	15	15
16	Liberia	22	17	14	17	17	17	16	16	15	21	15	17	17	18	18	15	17	17	16	17	16	17
17	Guinea	10	14	10	21	16	15	18	22	26	7	19	19	15	13	13	21	16	14	17	14	14	18
18	São Tomé and Príncipe	41	20	21	14	21	25	12	10	8	46	17	14	20	26	29	12	19	19	18	20	22	16
19	Sierra Leone	27	18	18	20	14	10	25	20	22	14	18	16	19	19	23	17	18	18	19	18	18	19
20	Burkina Faso	26	19	16	24	19	18	21	19	19	22	21	22	18	24	26	18	21	21	20	19	20	20
21	Comoros	19	22	26	15	20	20	22	18	18	28	20	21	22	22	25	20	20	20	21	21	21	21
22	Yemen	25	23	24	22	27	28	19	21	21	29	27	29	21	16	12	32	23	23	22	24	25	22
23	Eritrea	7	27	27	19	26	27	20	28	30	10	23	24	23	15	10	34	22	22	23	22	19	28
24	Togo	23	25	25	25	25	24	24	27	28	17	22	20	25	23	21	27	24	24	25	23	23	24
25	Mozambique	35	24	22	26	24	23	26	23	25	27	24	23	24	29	32	22	25	25	24	25	24	27

Table 4.3—Continued

Baseline Rank	Country or Territory	Unweighted (all weights = 1)	Demographic			Health Care			Public Health			Disease Dynamics			Political - Domestic			Political - International			Economic		
			Double	Triple	Zero	Double	Triple	Zero	Double	Triple	Zero	Double	Triple	Zero	Double	Triple	Zero	Double	Triple	Zero	Double	Triple	Zero
Not in Baseline, Top 25																							
46	Democratic People's Republic of Korea (North Korea)	3									24					24							
26	Republic of the Congo (Congo-Brazzaville)	15			23			23	24	24		25	25		21	20							23
30	Sudan	21									18				20	14							
28	Côte d'Ivoire	24	21	20		23	22				13												
27	Nigeria			23		22	21				20						24						25
29	Malawi								25	23							23						
58	Equatorial Guinea									13													
50	Cameroon										23												
39	Burundi										25												
51	Syria															22							
34	Senegal																25						

NOTE: Green cell = country originally among 25 most vulnerable, moved out of top 25; red cell = country originally not among top 25 most vulnerable, moved into top 25.

26), and Mozambique (25 to 35). Within the top 25, several countries increased in vulnerability (e.g., South Sudan, DRC, the Gambia, Guinea, Eritrea), while others fell to lower levels among the top 25. While all of these countries are no doubt highly vulnerable to infectious disease, the notable drop of seemingly more at-risk countries, such as Mauritania, Angola, and Afghanistan, suggest that our initial, subjective weighting better captured both the absolute and relative vulnerability of these countries—i.e., the baseline weighting scheme appeared to be a better reflection of risk than the completely unweighted scheme.

As shown in Table 4.3, the doubling, tripling, and zeroing out of each domain weight (which acted as a multiplier for the variable weights for the parameters within the domain) did little to change the composition of the top-25 most-vulnerable countries. Fourteen of the 16 most-vulnerable countries remained within the top 25 across all perturbations of domain weights. For the others, they mostly fell slightly out of the top 25 (seven of the 37 changes kept countries within the top-30 most vulnerable, replaced by countries for which baseline ranks were only slightly outside the top 25, with just a few exceptions). There were two particularly striking findings from our sensitivity analyses. First, no country fell out of the top-25 most vulnerable with doubling, tripling, or zeroing out the domain weight for the political-international domain, suggesting that this domain may contribute least to overall vulnerability. Second, zeroing out the public health domain weight resulted in the largest number of countries—six—falling out of the top 25, suggesting the greatest sensitivity to elimination of that domain from our algorithm. Otherwise, zeroing out other domain weights resulted in very little change to the top-25 most-vulnerable countries.

From these sensitivity tests, we concluded that the results are not strongly driven by a single factor or the further weight assigned to any specific domain. For the most part, the top-25 most-vulnerable countries remained in that range across each change in weighting values; the great majority of changes kept countries within the top-30 most vulnerable. Thus, the minimal variance resulting from our sensitivity testing would seem to validate the robustness of our tool and the resulting vulnerability scores.

Implications of the Findings

Our findings suggest that a broad range of factors collectively shapes a country's resilience to infectious diseases, rather than a single factor or domain alone. This first became evident while examining the connection between a country's overall vulnerability score to its levels of economic strength and development. Some countries outperformed their economic indicators—their overall normed vulnerability score was better (i.e., higher value) than their normed economic score alone might have predicted. A few of the 25 least-vulnerable (i.e., most resilient) countries were able to achieve this: Portugal and Japan in particular were more resilient than their economic domain scores alone might have suggested. For these two countries, the very positive score for the public health domain drove the overall score toward greater resilience. This indicates that the countries' health systems outperformed measures of income per capita and economic productivity in terms of predicting the degree of vulnerability to disease outbreaks. More relevant to the case of developing nations, however, may be the countries among the 50 most vulnerable for which the overall vulnerability scores were also substantially better than the economic domain scores, such as Eritrea (23), Malawi (29), Zimbabwe (35), Lesotho (38), and Burundi (39), among others. Table 4.4 presents the top-ten countries (among the 50 most vulnerable) that outperformed their economic domain score, as shown by the relatively large positive difference between the overall normed score and the economic domain score. The better overall vulnerability for most of these countries was driven more by the very low economic domain score rather than a consistently higher score in another specific domain. However, as with Portugal and Japan, the high (good) public health domain scores for Ethiopia and Cameroon drove up the overall vulnerability score (toward greater resilience and lower vulnerability). Vulnerable countries with weak health systems might look to these countries as examples of ways in which health systems were improved with relatively fewer resources, resulting in expectations for lower vulnerability to disease outbreaks.

Table 4.5 presents the bottom 11 countries, with the largest differences in the opposite direction—i.e., whose overall normed scores were even worse than predicted

Table 4.4
Countries Among Top 50 Most Vulnerable That Outperform Their Economic Indicators

Rank for Outperformance of Economic Domain Score	Country or Territory	Rank—Overall Vulnerability Score	Normed Overall Score	Normed Economic Domain Score	Difference Between Overall and Economic Domain Scores
1	Burundi	39	0.3541	0.0181	0.3360
2	Democratic People's Republic of Korea (North Korea)	46	0.3749	0.0901	0.2848
3	Eritrea	23	0.2530	0.0000	0.2530
4	Zimbabwe	35	0.3375	0.1024	0.2350
5	Rwanda	42	0.3553	0.1253	0.2300
6	Ethiopia	47	0.3820	0.1568	0.2253
7	Uganda	44	0.3659	0.1442	0.2216
8	Lesotho	38	0.3449	0.1247	0.2202
9	Cameroon	50	0.3888	0.1755	0.2133
10	Malawi	29	0.2800	0.0831	0.1969

Table 4.5
Countries That Most Underperform Their Economic Indicators

Rank for Outperformance of Economic Domain Score	Country or Territory	Rank—Overall Vulnerability Score	Normed Overall Score	Normed Economic Domain Score	Difference Between Overall and Economic Domain Scores
1	Brunei	159	0.7629	0.8742	−0.1114
2	Kuwait	131	0.6649	0.7724	−0.1076
3	United Arab Emirates	161	0.7652	0.8611	−0.0959
4	Equatorial Guinea	58	0.4301	0.5190	−0.0890
5	Luxembourg	177	0.8757	0.9627	−0.0870
6	Singapore	178	0.8783	0.9642	−0.0859
7	South Sudan	4	0.1008	0.1866	−0.0858
8	Turkmenistan	66	0.4867	0.5680	−0.0813
9	Somalia	1	0.0000	0.0757	−0.0757
10	Gabon	52	0.4030	0.4682	−0.0653
11	Taiwan	146	0.7097	0.7659	−0.0562

by their normed economic domain scores (differences in the negative direction). This list ranges from wealthy countries whose overall vulnerability scores did not match their economic scores (e.g., Brunei, Kuwait, United Arab Emirates, Luxembourg, Singapore) to poorer countries for which the noneconomic domains drove the vulnerability scores to even lower values, indicating greater vulnerability overall (e.g., Equatorial Guinea, South Sudan, Somalia, Gabon).

One important caveat that bears mention is that increased spending on public health, in the short run, that compromises long-run gains in economic growth and development could be detrimental to vulnerability to infectious disease in the future. If the public health sector is to be shored up so that current disease vulnerability is reduced, the government must try to do so in a way that does not compromise economic gains, which are also important to long-run resiliency.

Zika and Ebola as Empirical Examples

We examined the cases of the Zika virus in the Americas (2015–2016) and the Ebola virus in Africa (2014–2015) as empirical examples to assess the value and potential limitations of our Infectious Disease Vulnerability Index.

Zika virus spread rapidly across the Americas in 2015–2016, affecting all South American countries except Chile (which does not have the mosquito vector). By March 2016, Brazil and Colombia had reported the largest number of cases. Interestingly, results from our tool indicate that all South American countries outperformed their economic indicators—i.e., their overall vulnerability scores were better than what would have been predicted from their economic scores alone. While Brazil and Colombia do not necessarily stand out in terms of overall infectious disease vulnerability (as seen in Figure 4.3 and in the full scores reported in Appendix A), they both have certain factors that make them susceptible to a disease like the Zika virus. Zika flourishes in population-dense areas with abundant stagnant or standing water in which the disease-carrying mosquitoes can lay their eggs. In Brazil and Colombia, there are large urban slums that feature poor sanitation and hygiene conditions that are ripe for Zika to spread. Despite those countries' overall satisfactory performances in the tool, the high levels of inequality in Brazil and Colombia (both of which boast two of South America's highest Gini coefficients—a common measure for inequality within a given country) mean that health conditions and services vary widely within these countries. Our model does not evaluate income inequality within countries, so this may be a factor driving the rapid spread of the disease in underserved areas. In fact, both Brazil and Colombia score poorly for government service provision relative to the rest of South America. Poor service provision combined with high inequality and a fertile environment for a particular disease provide the conditions needed for a Zika virus outbreak.

The Zika virus example illustrates an important benefit of our tool as well as a limitation. The tool is designed to show vulnerability. That is, it will highlight which states are least likely to be able to cope with a serious disease outbreak within their country. It does not, however, strictly predict the likelihood of a disease arriving in a country or what will actually happen once it does arrive. Brazil and Colombia, because of unique economic and demographic challenges as well as the high prevalence of the mosquito vector, have experienced high numbers of Zika cases. West African countries were at greater risk for the spread of Ebola. What our model does show is which countries will be better placed to react to such risks—more resilient—and with what resources, though new diseases present new and different challenges, as the world health community witnessed with both the Ebola and Zika viruses.

We used the Ebola experience in West Africa as an empirical case to compare the three most-affected countries (Guinea, Liberia, Sierra Leone) with the four countries that more successfully contained the outbreak and limited the number of cases (Nigeria, DRC, Senegal, Mali), examining both the results from our algorithm and other factors that might have contributed to the outcomes observed. All three heavily affected countries and two of the four more-successful countries were among the 25 most-vulnerable countries (see Table 4.1: Nigeria ranked 27 and Senegal ranked 34).

Table 4.6 summarizes the key dates and number of cases for all seven African countries experiencing Ebola during 2014, listed in order of date of first reported case.

Figure 4.3
Map of Infectious Disease Vulnerability for Brazil and Its Neighbors

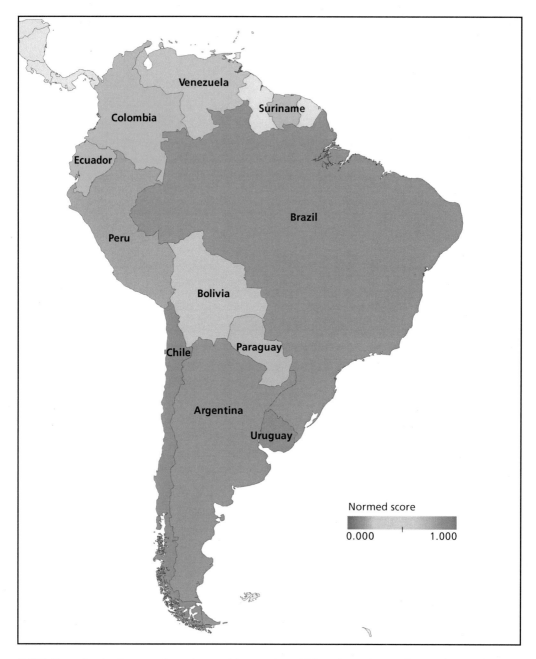

NOTE: The color shading runs from deep red (most vulnerable) to deeper green (least vulnerable).
RAND *RR1605-4.3*

Table 4.6
Outbreak Summary for the Seven African Countries Experiencing Ebola in 2014

Country	Date of First Case	Date Declared Ebola-Free	Total Cases	Total Deaths
Guinea	(December 2013) March 23, 2014	December 29, 2015	3,804	2,536
Liberia	March 29, 2014	January 14, 2016	19,675	4,808
Sierra Leone	May 25, 2014	March 17, 2016	14,122	3,955
Nigeria	July 23, 2014	October 20, 2014	20	8
Democratic Republic of the Congo	August 24, 2014	November 21, 2014	66	49
Senegal	August 29, 2014	October 17, 2014	1	0
Mali	October 23, 2014	January 18, 2015	8	6

SOURCE: CDC, 2016.

NOTE: The first case in Guinea occurred in December 2013 but was not recognized and diagnosed as Ebola until March 2014.

Of note, initial cases in Guinea, Liberia, and Sierra Leone preceded initial cases in the other four countries by at least two months. The WHO's declaration of Ebola as a public health emergency of international concern in early August 2014 preceded initial cases in three of those four countries (WHO, 2014a). Those countries might have been better sensitized to the possibility of Ebola and better able to respond quickly given the knowledge of the potential scope of the problem and the readiness of the international community to provide timely support. The later timing of cases in those countries might have contributed to their success with the Ebola outbreak, even though, according to our vulnerability index, they are among the most-vulnerable countries in the world.

Table 4.7 presents the outputs from our algorithm for these seven countries—the normed scores overall, the scores for each domain, and the scores that reflect countries' degrees of core public health capacity under the WHO's IHR. In line with the events as they unfolded during the Ebola 2014 outbreak, the average vulnerability rank for the three most heavily affected countries was 17, compared with 21 for the four more-successful countries. Across these seven countries, the three most heavily affected noticeably scored lower than the other four in the economic and political-international domains. The other domains, including health care, public health (including the composite IHR core capacity indicator), and political-domestic, did not neatly distinguish between the countries ultimately heavily affected by Ebola and those that more successfully responded in 2014. The timing of initial cases seems to best distinguish between the three heavily affected and four more-successful countries.

Table 4.7
Summary of Vulnerability Scores for African Countries Experiencing Ebola in 2014

Rank	Country or Territory	Overall	Demographic Domain	Health Care Domain	Public Health Domain	Disease Dynamic Domain	Political-Domestic Domain	Political-International Domain	Economic Domain	IHR Composite (factor score)
						Normed Score				
Heavily affected countries										
16	Liberia	0.2131	0.1962	0.2952	0.2980	0.3996	0.2429	0.3258	0.0958	0.5079
17	Guinea	0.2132	0.0692	0.2207	0.4222	0.6631	0.1821	0.1160	0.0242	0.5892
19	Sierra Leone	0.2234	0.2037	0.0556	0.3993	0.2549	0.2721	0.4294	0.1087	0.6882
More-successful countries										
11	Democratic Republic of the Congo	0.1818	0.3934	0.1213	0.3694	0.3789	0.1094	0.3681	0.0530	0.7118
12	Mali	0.1843	0.1792	0.1380	0.2497	0.4911	0.2494	0.4501	0.1496	0.5079
27	Nigeria	0.2707	0.3232	0.1887	0.4070	0.3137	0.2655	0.5422	0.2011	0.5686
34	Senegal	0.3292	0.1690	0.3633	0.3844	0.3619	0.4284	0.4952	0.1843	0.5975

NOTE: The color shading runs from deep red (most vulnerable) to deeper green (least vulnerable).

Interestingly, DRC and Mali, which were among the more-successful countries, appear to be more vulnerable than all three of the heavily affected countries. It is important to keep in mind, however, what the vulnerability index scores and rankings are meant to communicate. They are meant to indicate the level of vulnerability (or resilience) in a hypothetical scenario and suggest where extra effort might be needed to successfully address an infectious disease challenge, such as Ebola. They do not predict what will actually happen in the face of an outbreak. For example, DRC's success in containing the Ebola outbreak has been partly attributed to the robust and extensive response plans it already developed from its experiences with six previous outbreaks (WHO, 2014b). Nigeria's success came from several positive response elements, including prompt identification of the index case, strong government response, successful mobilization of internal and external funds, and effective coordination of response efforts (Chamberlin et al., 2015).

An interesting lesson from the examination of Ebola-affected countries in 2014 is that the expected level of vulnerability of a country does not sentence it to fail in controlling an infectious disease outbreak. Targeted, timely, and culturally sensitive interventions in public health, health care, incident management, and governance, as well as prompt global aid response, can help in mitigating an infectious disease outbreak, as seen in the examples of Nigeria, Senegal, and Mali (Chamberlin et al., 2015).

Furthermore, the success of a country during the recent Ebola outbreak is not necessarily a testament to the extent of the country's resilience. For example, while Nigeria successfully controlled the Ebola outbreak within three months, with a total of 20 deaths, it has more recently been battling another infectious hemorrhagic illness—Lassa fever. Although not as virulent as Ebola, more than 80 deaths were recorded between August 2015 and January 2016 (WHO, 2016). As discussed, while effective response interventions may help mitigate the spread of the outbreak, there may still be glaring vulnerabilities that our tool exposes systematically.

Hence, this tool is designed to be more of an aid to suggest countries that may be especially vulnerable and thus potential priorities for health engagement and capacity-building activities, such as training and equipping laboratories, strengthening biosurveillance, or pandemic preparedness exercises. The tool does not strictly predict success or failure in outbreak response.

CHAPTER FIVE
Conclusions and Next Steps

Because of the increasing risk to developing and developed countries alike posed by a range of infectious diseases, it is essential to have a clear understanding of current vulnerabilities at the country level across the globe—*where* the most-vulnerable countries are and *what* contributes most to their vulnerabilities. The Ebola crisis and the numerous infectious disease threats before it made it patently clear that infectious diseases do not respect political borders, nor do they remain contained in certain regions for very long in a hyper-connected world. RAND researchers developed the Infectious Disease Vulnerability Index as a tool to help identify countries that are potentially most vulnerable to poorly controlled infectious disease outbreaks because of a confluence of factors ranging across multiple domains, including political, economic, public health, medical, demographic, and disease dynamics. This information can help international actors—including bilateral, multilateral, and organizational partners—prioritize their respective programming to work with vulnerable countries to address weaknesses proactively, before problems emerge and get out of hand, and certainly to rally quickly to offer support to them when a disease threat does emerge. This report supports the recommendations of Gelfeld et al., 2015, in taking the next logical step to develop a more rigorously and quantitatively based tool to help assess the vulnerability and resilience of countries to infectious diseases. While the index cannot predict the occurrence or response to outbreaks, it does point to countries that are most vulnerable to such threats, for purposes of proactive programming to build country capabilities and the timely offering of support to response efforts once an outbreak emerges.

RAND recommends that DoD, HHS, other U.S. government agencies, and other international partners use this tool to inform their programming—to help identify vulnerable countries and set priorities for helping those countries build the capabilities they need to combat potential transnational disease outbreaks. As our results indicate, there are countries within certain regions that are more vulnerable, and the potential for infectious diseases to spread rapidly across highly vulnerable, contiguous countries merits serious attention. The "infectious disease belt" that stretches from West Africa to the Horn of Africa is particularly concerning.

The index highlights the connections between political stability and governance, economic development, and disease vulnerability. With this information in mind and by working with these and other vulnerable countries to improve health systems, governance, and development outcomes, the international community can help shore up the world's defenses against diseases and foster the cooperative and communicative networks that will lead to better, more-coordinated disease response. For example, the U.S. government and its associated departments and agencies (e.g., DoD, USAID, and HHS, including the CDC) can work with governments of states that are particularly vulnerable in order to improve their public health systems (e.g., disease surveillance, laboratory testing, outbreak detection, rapid response teams for investigation and disease control measures) and medical care systems (e.g., professional training and certification, clinic and hospital care). Aid organizations such as USAID also support economic development and efforts to strengthen governance. For example, better governance through democracy-promotion and anticorruption programs may lead to less vulnerability as states improve coordination, communication, and infrastructure systems that help to combat infectious disease transmission. Finally, exercises, including tabletop exercises, can be used to help countries better understand actions and actors, and the coordination needed among them, to best prepare their systems to respond effectively to a disease threat that arises.

Given that resources for such endeavors are often scarce, we should take lessons from countries whose disease resilience has outperformed their level of economic development to find cost-effective, context-appropriate solutions that will work in these challenging environments. In Rwanda, for example, improved governance and administration of aid, alongside reduced corruption, has allowed for higher vaccination rates and greater investment in public health and community health care services (Hamblin, 2014).

While we have shown that this tool is robust to significant changes in weights across all domains, we designed it to be interactive: End users can change the weights to reflect their beliefs or changing realities on the ground. The Infectious Disease Vulnerability Index is intended to inform actions addressing infectious disease preparedness and response to foster greater resiliency of national, regional, and global systems. We have already witnessed the devastating results of a reactive approach to infectious disease control during the Ebola crisis. The international community would do well to take more-extensive, preemptive measures to address the vulnerability at the country level in advance of future disease crises.

Overall Country Rankings

Table A.1 presents, in ranked order, the normed overall scores for the 195 countries examined, from most vulnerable (i.e., lowest score) to least vulnerable (highest score). The color shading runs from deep red (most vulnerable) through orange and yellow to light and deeper green (least vulnerable).

Table A.1
Overall Country Rankings

Rank	Country or Territory	Combatant Command	Overall Score Normed	Demographic Domain Score	Health Care Domain Score	Public Health Domain Score	Disease Dynamics Domain Score	Political-Domestic Domain Score	Political-International Domain Score	Economic Domain Score
1	Somalia	AFRICOM	0.000000	0.348761269	0.058301438	0	0.629775134	0	0.102936726	0.075656481
2	Central African Republic	AFRICOM	0.000061	0.15529298	0	0.045046954	0.548852541	0.053250913	0.315859162	0.005423805
3	Chad	AFRICOM	0.098450	0.21024639	0.049051336	0.18881211	0.543405231	0.115586538	0.259990693	0.10676029
4	South Sudan	AFRICOM	0.100836	0.007304932	0.231601644	0.18968877	0.415040266	0.084988387	0.355877361	0.186605024
5	Mauritania	AFRICOM	0.107294	0.303529503	0.20019796	0.013730395	0.542586879	0.19966007	0.267845057	0.219330172
6	Angola	AFRICOM	0.148414	0.482859258	0.00080090	0.164124037	0.733107108	0.186137702	0.368890955	0.15088322
7	Haiti	SOUTHCOM	0.149471	0.338437297	0.301310943	0.18504928	0.50577236	0.126225355	0.400839569	0.082264511
8	Afghanistan	CENTCOM	0.157034	0.151637325	0.199607537	0.326981557	0.707856514	0.073169519	0.362626952	0.077103098
9	Niger	AFRICOM	0.166531	0	0.254825107	0.193413572	0.573089179	0.269691628	0.412882392	0.095023518
10	Madagascar	AFRICOM	0.170787	0.472647362	0.40269105	0.038220819	0.345020655	0.313366918	0.161904122	0.020461077
11	Democratic Republic of the Congo	AFRICOM	0.18762	0.393402129	0.12133578	0.369430992	0.378852278	0.10394181	0.368097103	0.052965522
12	Mali	AFRICOM	0.184254	0.179173821	0.138023501	0.2496769	0.49111854	0.249390347	0.450073263	0.149625848
13	Guinea-Bissau	AFRICOM	0.187841	0.306480143	0.25150669	0.283305699	0.347653436	0.18650838	0.309947808	0.077079134
14	Benin	AFRICOM	0.206682	0.102429204	0.205857213	0.198587465	0.411218562	0.375126664	0.461867546	0.132700537
15	The Gambia	AFRICOM	0.207809	0.223431605	0.330645436	0.250325387	0.531156832	0.250433571	0.26696682	0.074090725
16	Liberia	AFRICOM	0.213114	0.196208895	0.295150785	0.298018392	0.399575501	0.24289448	0.325809636	0.095770949

Table A.1—Continued

Rank	Country or Territory	Combatant Command	Overall Score Normed	Demographic Domain Score	Health Care Domain Score	Public Health Domain Score	Disease Dynamics Domain Score	Political-Domestic Domain Score	Political-International Domain Score	Economic Domain Score
17	Guinea	AFRICOM	0.213225	0.069168696	0.220723728	0.422224209	0.663071602	0.18076736	0.116032771	0.024189584
18	São Tomé and Príncipe	AFRICOM	0.223256	0.456315076	0.45499994	0.08756294	0.199137462	0.337999767	0.441651348	0.198939704
19	Sierra Leone	AFRICOM	0.223397	0.20367201	0.055611728	0.399252552	0.254903955	0.272075698	0.429440571	0.108721252
20	Burkina Faso	AFRICOM	0.231504	0.141437335	0.237090446	0.292575172	0.677980032	0.291887418	0.60014903	0.105762283
21	Comoros	AFRICOM	0.238068	0.54485136	0.275448866	0.252023099	0.444342284	0.267647568	0.225866673	0.111809438
22	Yemen	CENTCOM	0.250277	0.433731647	0.431651802	0.332075013	0.800080626	0.104453177	0.284363402	0.21272156
23	Eritrea	AFRICOM	0.252978	0.514020768	0.410049982	0.45304433	0.482945814	0.0855761	0.09121531	0
24	Togo	AFRICOM	0.259396	0.405922983	0.301568399	0.417204432	0.154799483	0.210826371	0.273656224	0.115077926
25	Mozambique	AFRICOM	0.262501	0.359585689	0.260453468	0.332816947	0.316911572	0.313880616	0.463545305	0.108794995
26	Republic of the Congo (Congo-Brazzaville)	AFRICOM	0.268887	0.570590666	0.437612936	0.316875454	0.28890352	0.178093753	0.30517259	0.252505538
27	Nigeria	AFRICOM	0.270681	0.323201474	0.188728449	0.407012765	0.313685957	0.265472276	0.542161976	0.201149401
28	Côte d'Ivoire	AFRICOM	0.270743	0.149916663	0.198317769	0.480959396	0.293965416	0.244095631	0.2675316	0.21451864
29	Malawi	AFRICOM	0.279987	0.458224208	0.358702184	0.288097304	0.339690734	0.3511682	0.388453718	0.083074415
30	Sudan	AFRICOM	0.291580	0.588865802	0.33955302	0.494972938	0.568033919	0.08367456	0.236802875	0.173847044
31	Djibouti	AFRICOM	0.297892	0.516489993	0.308140349	0.360228068	0.494501563	0.275017476	0.461575379	0.186799289
32	Pakistan	CENTCOM	0.308544	0.356313929	0.199267938	0.433297664	0.534440723	0.284108175	0.399359647	0.292054119

Table A.1—Continued

Rank	Country or Territory	Combatant Command	Overall Score Normed	Demographic Domain Score	Health Care Domain Score	Public Health Domain Score	Disease Dynamics Domain Score	Political-Domestic Domain Score	Political-International Domain Score	Economic Domain Score
33	Timor-Leste	PACOM	0.310208	0.479566717	0.363006819	0.402401796	0.379571232	0.253405013	0.287238579	0.252405183
34	Senegal	AFRICOM	0.329156	0.16895548	0.363332743	0.384433278	0.361880002	0.428403911	0.495175169	0.184325671
35	Zimbabwe	AFRICOM	0.337478	0.697284238	0.343816002	0.485627407	0.653775962	0.199349794	0.410356268	0.102445378
36	Papua New Guinea	PACOM	0.339184	0.525901322	0.358755958	0.461298605	0.131831164	0.302787534	0.350931307	0.206087372
37	Tanzania	AFRICOM	0.340445	0.515884251	0.42046585	0.37514479	0.404598376	0.346796951	0.569472596	0.15939076
38	Lesotho	AFRICOM	0.344860	0.699269239	0.193535354	0.381086761	0.494889941	0.403306048	0.485893078	0.124695851
39	Burundi	AFRICOM	0.354104	0.677770717	0.28284965	0.595976924	0.446364064	0.21929185	0.278333482	0.018062778
40	Laos	PACOM	0.355111	0.617197869	0.303718578	0.470396949	0.316874844	0.303216875	0.335972175	0.244014369
41	Cambodia	PACOM	0.355133	0.603977974	0.501870948	0.389329462	0.249954709	0.30794789	0.347829899	0.26833912
42	Rwanda	AFRICOM	0.355300	0.485789716	0.462248927	0.428403858	0.316105011	0.352489703	0.416536032	0.125261052
43	Swaziland	AFRICOM	0.358470	0.753558504	0.380812489	0.443187479	0.218933247	0.269991159	0.555068926	0.244366007
44	Uganda	AFRICOM	0.365850	0.588681047	0.41351401	0.458546659	0.373898751	0.333622855	0.332674624	0.144241411
45	Solomon Islands	PACOM	0.370311	0.707450052	0.534428456	0.37671347	0	0.373395199	0.467899811	0.179128527
46	Democratic People's Republic of Korea (North Korea)	PACOM	0.374870	0.907296141	0.613281963	0.586079979	0.611464602	0.054304985	0	0.090100341
47	Ethiopia	AFRICOM	0.382021	0.28569545	0.39330463	0.622299852	0.499217243	0.272946162	0.492468433	0.156768353

Table A.1—Continued

Rank	Country or Territory	Combatant Command	Overall Score Normed	Demographic Domain Score	Health Care Domain Score	Public Health Domain Score	Disease Dynamics Domain Score	Political-Domestic Domain Score	Political-International Domain Score	Economic Domain Score
48	Kenya	AFRICOM	0.385436	0.610453351	0.415088725	0.489142677	0.406130325	0.316426717	0.518261714	0.20694373
49	Kiribati	PACOM	0.388403	0.654475766	0.488085296	0.405577185	0.297866678	0.385759659	0.475592649	0.205151343
50	Cameroon	AFRICOM	0.388770	0.51903402	0.258084837	0.695554838	0.464468675	0.203603511	0.493377384	0.175481005
51	Syria	CENTCOM	0.391337	0.766302674	0.625200685	0.600996701	0.624323285	0.04013296	0.300755443	0.284843637
52	Gabon	AFRICOM	0.402950	0.607270396	0.461092427	0.411908948	0.391552681	0.347626656	0.507560675	0.468207358
53	Nepal	PACOM	0.404405	0.43755136	0.45526256	0.61031371	0.463079764	0.278476918	0.285340204	0.207989533
54	Honduras	SOUTHCOM	0.407296	0.65516817	0.568583253	0.402040524	0.401156848	0.371453871	0.548887432	0.271822983
55	Zambia	AFRICOM	0.420459	0.43163488	0.365427589	0.580965131	0.520140049	0.388834572	0.589087275	0.160896589
56	Bangladesh	PACOM	0.422107	0.406154362	0.441798669	0.695174552	0.461126045	0.259707056	0.364340005	0.176276411
57	Micronesia	PACOM	0.425305	0.618409374	0.547928079	0.460395425	0.5414935	0.423698655	0.04691838	0.167555551
58	Equatorial Guinea	AFRICOM	0.430054	0.86324907	0.211610892	0.637801825	0.400635817	0.215602062	0.220558685	0.519011312
59	Iraq	CENTCOM	0.432182	0.503984852	0.515920977	0.701934137	0.502859325	0.168166417	0.402990831	0.320138576
60	Myanmar	PACOM	0.448176	0.77384107	0.379347207	0.807929378	0.379456154	0.137665674	0.213666835	0.225276745
61	Palestine	CENTCOM	0.450415	0.7436505	0.501813229	0.642310982	0.604772521	0.248676492	0.261521404	0.223952424
62	Bhutan	PACOM	0.460880	0.452080334	0.483140955	0.488859839	0.605787331	0.490043329	0.262023123	0.356907842
63	Ghana	AFRICOM	0.462565	0.526023873	0.370472249	0.543649558	0.431181585	0.500767939	0.616686004	0.248491531
64	Guatemala	SOUTHCOM	0.477179	0.628594639	0.518759849	0.579187293	0.575328055	0.367784506	0.52762574	0.347084061
65	Cape Verde	AFRICOM	0.486189	0.631853881	0.535080169	0.462030655	0.475776594	0.521787662	0.538518732	0.347072706

Table A.1—Continued

Rank	Country or Territory	Combatant Command	Overall Score Normed	Demographic Domain Score	Health Care Domain Score	Public Health Domain Score	Disease Dynamics Domain Score	Political-Domestic Domain Score	Political-International Domain Score	Economic Domain Score
66	Turkmenistan	CENTCOM	0.486696	0.866733101	0.50185344	0.662080155	0.675431715	0.177345824	0.245358453	0.567962822
67	Namibia	AFRICOM	0.490478	0.728321661	0.471954399	0.44645794	0.578010862	0.523755903	0.672243408	0.370783642
68	Vanuatu	PACOM	0.490878	0.716342676	0.548938734	0.533251326	0.828054424	0.436297938	0.424226226	0.217200362
69	Nicaragua	SOUTHCOM	0.492491	0.638084587	0.566071409	0.660197738	0.232783952	0.364495143	0.442663666	0.291765645
70	Libya	AFRICOM	0.493272	0.874139158	0.677912554	0.690021675	0.905000916	0.13026655	0.266478037	0.354558564
71	India	PACOM	0.493799	0.527272726	0.411687541	0.611043384	0.442952339	0.47193106	0.549585696	0.342247507
72	Algeria	AFRICOM	0.496612	0.706981418	0.558980692	0.611159847	0.656533024	0.317721818	0.398632623	0.437323933
73	Dominican Republic	SOUTHCOM	0.499533	0.651841382	0.52728257	0.561931812	0.34117008	0.41008651	0.751048964	0.487357273
74	Jamaica	SOUTHCOM	0.499783	0.803953609	0.589106624	0.466499017	0.197174286	0.474726908	0.544630277	0.474210427
75	Bolivia	SOUTHCOM	0.500436	0.783350995	0.46887641	0.550798937	0.609031246	0.436445721	0.483681062	0.35940819
76	Tajikistan	CENTCOM	0.507026	0.864911268	0.485530073	0.713000462	0.907404316	0.237810489	0.349216002	0.317040961
77	Uzbekistan	CENTCOM	0.515492	0.921624713	0.576668339	0.664856243	0.853273942	0.245043684	0.310194908	0.383443552
78	Saint Lucia	SOUTHCOM	0.516511	0.810879343	0.612550332	0.411353459	0.410794853	0.562974621	0.909730849	0.359239928
79	Bosnia and Herzegovina	EUCOM	0.523079	0.913672874	0.730287281	0.477584357	0.328960513	0.4335209	0.438477804	0.457486886
80	Egypt	CENTCOM	0.530405	0.618601857	0.592082614	0.772762422	0.790643968	0.241970707	0.566291639	0.396148261
81	Venezuela	SOUTHCOM	0.530692	0.897045602	0.619258291	0.690349672	0.39175468	0.30915459	0.210215036	0.383245346
82	Tunisia	AFRICOM	0.535451	0.69601836	0.63618194	0.554231019	0.776448056	0.434017521	0.545007557	0.450207048
83	Paraguay	SOUTHCOM	0.541167	0.887420329	0.585820732	0.596008162	0.34557185	0.438463994	0.514414762	0.408028299

Table A.1—Continued

Rank	Country or Territory	Combatant Command	Overall Score Normed	Demographic Domain Score	Health Care Domain Score	Public Health Domain Score	Disease Dynamics Domain Score	Political-Domestic Domain Score	Political-International Domain Score	Economic Domain Score
84	Marshall Islands	PACOM	0.544611	0.733122429	0.56898489	0.709406759	0.48890968	0.377615668	0.356184447	0.384185218
85	Philippines	PACOM	0.544923	0.77982774	0.569482929	0.6075091	0.335072899	0.486973807	0.50580298	0.374891865
86	Lebanon	CENTCOM	0.546332	0.795573254	0.703444198	0.598116034	0.671265282	0.359178936	0.531402066	0.496274896
87	Botswana	AFRICOM	0.548363	0.754044035	0.454855452	0.498290934	0.47607347	0.614109149	0.66328916	0.470789877
88	Saint Vincent and the Grenadines	SOUTHCOM	0.549145	0.819932978	0.602106622	0.471895005	0.372237992	0.594954664	0.607374498	0.41767656
89	Azerbaijan	EUCOM	0.550328	0.80274177	0.599807177	0.698233478	0.606958685	0.32056515	0.454723753	0.487222886
90	Belize	SOUTHCOM	0.551546	0.771835129	0.602063419	0.649761602	0.463750568	0.486547326	0.705431728	0.181641854
91	Guyana	SOUTHCOM	0.554987	0.891131054	0.458067511	0.708627172	0.296047164	0.416718306	0.628370039	0.391547761
92	Suriname	SOUTHCOM	0.555320	0.954190989	0.606685909	0.590168054	0.174932096	0.452661043	0.598203123	0.470173357
93	Kyrgyzstan	CENTCOM	0.555486	0.938771283	0.631595746	0.699298755	0.586997287	0.34098018	0.335903245	0.331551371
94	Indonesia	PACOM	0.562944	0.750619361	0.51111275	0.710992077	0.15555375	0.478663061	0.445239925	0.395961649
95	Fiji	PACOM	0.567238	0.912372761	0.550048845	0.793183785	0.338759095	0.315685028	0.457442072	0.404795695
96	Iran	CENTCOM	0.567841	0.784483428	0.612522278	0.882104181	0.624311112	0.198250398	0.230460389	0.442781114
97	Serbia	EUCOM	0.568934	0.916239959	0.722244933	0.499384257	0.480581894	0.51660661	0.405971768	0.4936118
98	Morocco	AFRICOM	0.569769	0.434646778	0.528876434	0.84548263	0.577067854	0.391024483	0.482941077	0.379778141
99	Sri Lanka	PACOM	0.571001	0.824058144	0.711895651	0.665711887	0.324270477	0.403023718	0.408839796	0.464799504
100	Ecuador	SOUTHCOM	0.575843	0.722701117	0.595184777	0.707058492	0.678173471	0.428549787	0.427197843	0.405811804

Table A.1—Continued

Rank	Country or Territory	Combatant Command	Overall Score Normed	Demographic Domain Score	Health Care Domain Score	Public Health Domain Score	Disease Dynamics Domain Score	Political-Domestic Domain Score	Political-International Domain Score	Economic Domain Score
101	Maldives	PACOM	0.576299	0.841874404	0.71580204	0.615057779	0.499207759	0.42243462	0.365921875	0.541604906
102	Samoa	PACOM	0.580679	0.921508717	0.592935194	0.676569055	0.366383014	0.490973549	0.632269107	0.264505253
103	Colombia	SOUTHCOM	0.583850	0.73590202	0.612534314	0.707762022	0.22902618	0.45935057	0.601974629	0.47801846
104	Trinidad and Tobago	SOUTHCOM	0.594998	0.891388245	0.593781874	0.588209581	0.297889543	0.52303962	0.702753024	0.620994685
105	Grenada	SOUTHCOM	0.597669	0.813492271	0.65338997	0.65938284	0.327863202	0.505583618	0.655573334	0.450723518
106	Kosovo	EUCOM	0.599085	0.812337384	0.64667112	0.700404301	0.948019768	0.421397702	0.297036976	0.43229239
107	Dominica	SOUTHCOM	0.604170	0.844714809	0.627354831	0.609489644	0.372910612	0.571179399	0.505129227	0.4850104
108	Panama	SOUTHCOM	0.606521	0.737928024	0.635029055	0.68180749	0.106062488	0.525841004	0.496356941	0.588123724
109	Kazakhstan	CENTCOM	0.607098	0.981048407	0.707658405	0.677881042	0.93945835	0.333781992	0.488876147	0.590940265
110	El Salvador	SOUTHCOM	0.607731	0.6191346	0.601234082	0.850540435	0.28724289	0.436493199	0.54421992	0.395198532
111	Tuvalu	PACOM	0.608741	0.875628325	0.618086156	0.755212219	0.642248938	0.444856565	0.25861146	0.363272122
112	Montenegro	EUCOM	0.612065	0.93168502	0.738004329	0.460452468	0.680756338	0.614974382	0.754847687	0.537121927
113	Belarus	EUCOM	0.616419	0.948117465	0.853060744	0.737852159	0.729005525	0.28632401	0.339082773	0.558616977
114	Ukraine	EUCOM	0.617343	0.936893751	0.758059683	0.74616146	0.502357605	0.369668189	0.517646543	0.470738673
115	Andorra	EUCOM	0.625221	0.899070911	0.81185289	0.335756658	0.630062854	0.739533878	0.766592386	0.626926946
116	Vietnam	PACOM	0.626124	0.768735331	0.591621982	0.904871434	0.41531068	0.382561816	0.423894556	0.399912654
117	Mongolia	PACOM	0.626185	0.852084539	0.64245526	0.666272809	0.870250764	0.510046178	0.53128146	0.471441687
118	Albania	EUCOM	0.626259	0.904696069	0.63796023	0.722971737	0.521323721	0.475157221	0.762993915	0.441433481

Table A.1—Continued

Rank	Country or Territory	Combatant Command	Overall Score Normed	Demographic Domain Score	Health Care Domain Score	Public Health Domain Score	Disease Dynamics Domain Score	Political-Domestic Domain Score	Political-International Domain Score	Economic Domain Score
119	Seychelles	AFRICOM	0.628108	0.810980857	0.657086791	0.687787494	0.390390083	0.494835838	0.518962829	0.655611717
120	Tonga	PACOM	0.630046	0.906132187	0.608256509	0.743499407	0.844821936	0.458585145	0.731682013	0.385257601
121	Oman	CENTCOM	0.633743	0.748969293	0.678305802	0.723211144	0.593656334	0.476394997	0.477227234	0.605681428
122	Mauritius	AFRICOM	0.635763	0.778503617	0.647800239	0.590301155	0.187100393	0.679208505	0.575721312	0.580459506
123	Moldova	EUCOM	0.635987	0.917660729	0.71345235	0.709739509	0.675492376	0.472488646	0.533946795	0.449328928
124	Russia	EUCOM	0.639878	0.805597169	0.79116595	0.738755338	0.863995549	0.395174473	0.359128816	0.582180922
125	Peru	SOUTHCOM	0.645670	0.735230187	0.612136964	0.815447159	0.492648593	0.499915615	0.596351721	0.451805721
126	Bahamas	NORTHCOM	0.653653	0.918739251	0.703075636	0.575317882	0.492042096	0.645633246	0.777444015	0.553475774
127	Romania	EUCOM	0.657694	0.927839309	0.716370279	0.589635654	0.699722172	0.587542888	0.905312991	0.600400812
128	Palau	PACOM	0.658010	0.940352086	0.669390872	0.773473082	0.563826585	0.461056723	0.513559461	0.550854819
129	China	PACOM	0.663535	0.803222219	0.660649638	0.912458141	0.727148738	0.347275227	0.771275554	0.524788199
130	Bahrain	CENTCOM	0.663702	0.798762025	0.689760115	0.786015392	0.664865855	0.408603355	0.506871008	0.783172021
131	Kuwait	CENTCOM	0.664856	0.81917289	0.713447831	0.766335587	0.667078749	0.419269242	0.524728011	0.77242657
132	Cyprus	EUCOM	0.665630	0.902755729	0.754888296	0.540426633	0.609054819	0.645857231	0.865849429	0.662576695
133	Bulgaria	EUCOM	0.666120	0.925371964	0.743478619	0.559307838	0.896878102	0.602198036	0.982629857	0.612549843
134	Turkey	EUCOM	0.677438	0.84102406	0.648323142	0.81050344	0.5061117	0.537330939	0.262969703	0.541217747
135	Barbados	SOUTHCOM	0.681515	0.859280737	0.659994467	0.636234961	0.433450974	0.702895509	0.697763236	0.565336196
136	Macedonia (FYROM)	EUCOM	0.685990	0.90279095	0.749151161	0.84972282	0.322258652	0.471897252	0.458219533	0.536808101

Table A.1—Continued

Rank	Country or Territory	Combatant Command	Overall Score Normed	Demographic Domain Score	Health Care Domain Score	Public Health Domain Score	Disease Dynamics Domain Score	Political-Domestic Domain Score	Political-International Domain Score	Economic Domain Score
137	San Marino	EUCOM	0.687314	0.877776833	0.836135825	0.561149509	0.518312718	0.679742104	0.766592386	0.64448737
138	Saint Kitts and Nevis	SOUTHCOM	0.691572	0.881290256	0.712891102	0.657549997	0.346677987	0.665293245	0.829339569	0.62074865
139	Antigua and Barbuda	SOUTHCOM	0.693938	0.893937326	0.667623825	0.743665782	0.245617562	0.63821691	0.520411413	0.575972221
140	Cuba	SOUTHCOM	0.695910	0.933526344	0.855484713	0.90303893	0.366456933	0.404214354	0.449537038	0.475762057
141	South Africa	AFRICOM	0.697292	0.739000698	0.492333001	0.910898968	0.728928869	0.555658151	0.806992812	0.458012442
142	Malta	EUCOM	0.706869	0.805461701	0.786086898	0.663106927	0.732150286	0.6068915	0.969012043	0.726319966
143	Armenia	EUCOM	0.706912	0.927925843	0.673316098	0.895147994	0.863693546	0.465782742	0.483460443	0.470591816
144	Argentina	SOUTHCOM	0.707041	0.948178606	0.691269478	0.808518822	0.560647472	0.553572732	0.556525845	0.541805549
145	Jordan	CENTCOM	0.707361	0.839002213	0.641234998	0.970736985	0.578743881	0.448303847	0.57726 1141	0.487309358
146	Taiwan	PACOM	0.709691	0.882856201	0.70431 2641	0.68002837	0.456275152	0.664178777	0.296789098	0.765940269
147	Thailand	PACOM	0.711334	0.885465372	0.62677221	0.962427734	0.62694065	0.437138287	0.727455976	0.521104959
148	Brazil	SOUTHCOM	0.716641	0.872669567	0.679129575	0.891725419	0.354111322	0.549222249	0.754472248	0.490921248
149	Croatia	EUCOM	0.719996	0.931182251	0.775185048	0.677605334	0.542865728	0.66604141 6	0.690373454	0.629194341
150	Greece	EUCOM	0.734145	0.906991647	0.761757264	0.732615619	0.376826734	0.648846923	0.916531927	0.688365064
151	Mexico	NORTHCOM	0.734971	0.895687193	0.681337082	0.929552001	0.484941568	0.543189203	0.602271831	0.501174898
152	Georgia	EUCOM	0.735821	0.932877706	0.688075552	0.933449934	0.67798806	0.521299946	0.557664397	0.459684241
153	Saudi Arabia	CENTCOM	0.736844	0.874779695	0.658704202	0.990759048	1	0.366061648	0.550754044	0.733411275

Table A.1—Continued

Rank	Country or Territory	Combatant Command	Overall Score Normed	Demographic Domain Score	Health Care Domain Score	Public Health Domain Score	Disease Dynamics Domain Score	Political-Domestic Domain Score	Political-International Domain Score	Economic Domain Score
154	Costa Rica	SOUTHCOM	0.736960	0.894380479	0.653306234	0.87446043	0.362911742	0.620583237	0.660345256	0.534136689
155	Liechtenstein	EUCOM	0.737219	0.896106283	0.815727483	0.586614417	0.827747953	0.758091292	0.766592386	0.659550605
156	Uruguay	SOUTHCOM	0.745957	0.950686562	0.740102998	0.662935798	0.438108226	0.773395983	0.909711237	0.607551891
157	Monaco	EUCOM	0.753737	0.791810891	1	0.677690899	0.651556882	0.679101567	0.766592386	0.660443708
158	Malaysia	PACOM	0.761135	0.839176914	0.67687186	0.875655955	0.493083835	0.63334295	0.668769102	0.673280121
159	Brunei	PACOM	0.762886	0.874687416	0.70489492	0.786619347	0.634752678	0.641875771	0.431018613	0.874246619
160	Latvia	EUCOM	0.763937	0.968617001	0.741818065	0.739791618	0.563571802	0.688153452	1	0.698508767
161	United Arab Emirates	CENTCOM	0.765200	0.847993152	0.716624307	0.804181184	0.598809732	0.636140693	0.520400766	0.861066271
162	Lithuania	EUCOM	0.771597	0.958628438	0.814773789	0.657041364	0.649251562	0.75532868	0.934379272	0.72347797
163	Israel	EUCOM	0.782439	0.854886204	0.770973902	0.919499772	0.600759896	0.581279009	0.379613864	0.747078747
164	Poland	EUCOM	0.782799	0.923971091	0.762207361	0.741059789	0.631680687	0.736503575	0.916531927	0.712935199
165	Qatar	CENTCOM	0.787534	0.825534433	0.859447393	0.815278407	0.532726357	0.591668269	0.604075439	1
166	Hungary	EUCOM	0.795623	0.918277432	0.780860606	0.795341909	0.612665331	0.718660223	0.74874504	0.716600159
167	Estonia	EUCOM	0.797443	0.961311269	0.788655215	0.747311775	0.650866111	0.740860321	0.916531927	0.733650967
168	Chile	SOUTHCOM	0.801129	0.928226436	0.659547664	0.826950813	0.672161075	0.774959487	0.653402606	0.633205173
169	Slovenia	EUCOM	0.805790	0.924463067	0.800752319	0.699680942	0.673445333	0.811944312	0.930263357	0.75096352
170	Slovakia	EUCOM	0.808457	0.919371646	0.773671333	0.804174053	0.62721411	0.738761446	0.916531927	0.71531865
171	Italy	EUCOM	0.821690	0.856231713	0.788830593	0.880230796	0.656117184	0.699986858	0.916531927	0.726620448

Table A.1—Continued

Rank	Country or Territory	Combatant Command	Overall Score Normed	Demographic Domain Score	Health Care Domain Score	Public Health Domain Score	Disease Dynamics Domain Score	Political-Domestic Domain Score	Political-International Domain Score	Economic Domain Score
172	Czech Republic	EUCOM	0.847175	0.906329381	0.858137428	0.841888926	0.675622303	0.758476946	0.916531927	0.754722666
173	France	EUCOM	0.855407	0.901560479	0.762328175	0.857658915	0.421396909	0.830016223	0.916531927	0.777041464
174	Belgium	EUCOM	0.870933	0.890373515	0.881717583	0.795398952	0.494758354	0.87486074	0.832638483	0.819913866
175	Austria	EUCOM	0.874243	0.918195691	0.839263106	0.734866913	0.711301404	0.928260114	0.916531927	0.824196757
176	Spain	EUCOM	0.875475	0.894413692	0.802359453	0.961553076	0.489746511	0.753628505	0.916531927	0.776630305
177	Luxembourg	EUCOM	0.875694	0.887993297	0.823089445	0.739297246	0.42133064	0.932009579	0.916531927	0.962689426
178	Singapore	PACOM	0.878289	0.75400878	0.758425964	0.883394777	0.383877239	0.86306891	0.766592386	0.964234101
179	Republic of Korea (South Korea)	PACOM	0.879402	0.877557638	0.770987107	0.995797839	0.461237065	0.772828274	0.497064669	0.773109163
180	Portugal	EUCOM	0.888782	0.876638524	0.79732637	0.958073458	0.50904535	0.82395019	0.916531927	0.704209425
181	United Kingdom	EUCOM	0.897495	0.873066095	0.791637218	0.903418741	0.405362686	0.880595772	0.916531927	0.834119172
182	Ireland	EUCOM	0.906320	0.934977624	0.840624597	0.848802528	0.61732229	0.882121273	0.916531927	0.891881987
183	Iceland	EUCOM	0.908112	1	0.858141488	0.827476084	0.668434151	0.918590951	0.74874504	0.79396266
184	Australia	PACOM	0.912517	0.975157866	0.812116885	0.870293921	0.47345486	0.924097329	0.74874504	0.827583221
185	Switzerland	EUCOM	0.915839	0.890580942	0.772600784	0.801310024	0.70225779	1	0.74874504	0.894005898
186	New Zealand	PACOM	0.916279	0.954940122	0.795754437	0.818929154	0.808190216	0.962851573	0.916531927	0.80260938
187	Netherlands	EUCOM	0.918935	0.887076534	0.73337715	0.920957536	0.553404325	0.917862548	0.916531927	0.862303793

Table A.1—Continued

Rank	Country or Territory	Combatant Command	Overall Score Normed	Demographic Domain Score	Health Care Domain Score	Public Health Domain Score	Disease Dynamics Domain Score	Political-Domestic Domain Score	Political-International Domain Score	Economic Domain Score
188	United States	NORTHCOM	0.924939	0.796419884	0.800665522	0.97031867	0.377648988	0.895287308	0.915531927	0.876147651
189	Japan	PACOM	0.926410	0.891150261	0.808687785	0.971763758	0.493467108	0.903673298	0.580958154	0.777210348
190	Denmark	EUCOM	0.953641	0.916586212	0.880801307	0.903844661	0.612908784	0.959806464	0.916531927	0.8538081
191	Sweden	EUCOM	0.955625	0.949114755	0.76126462	0.942120457	0.786708122	0.954243778	0.74874504	0.856365
192	Germany	EUCOM	0.966890	0.890219438	0.868542466	0.995094309	0.60005594	0.911542581	0.916531927	0.863184603
193	Finland	EUCOM	0.968274	0.965048379	0.836351059	0.915424373	0.862049549	0.988425759	0.74874504	0.810382184
194	Canada	NORTHCOM	0.973400	0.96349958 3	0.772758496	0.997414055	0.718699352	0.945881533	0.916531927	0.826922627
195	Norway	EUCOM	1	0.961329861	0.898074321	1	0.592155487	0.956851809	0.74874504	0.928046396

NOTE: The color shading runs from deep red (most vulnerable) through orange and yellow to light and deeper green (least vulnerable).

Country Bins for Missing Data Imputation

Table B.1 classifies the 195 countries we examined by income group and region, as defined by the World Bank. Missing data for a country were imputed using conditional means within the country's region-income group category. Colors in the bin, country or territory, and income group columns reflect the income group; colors in the combatant command and region classification columns reflect the DoD combatant command and World Bank region.

Table B.1
Country Subgroups Classified by World Bank Income Group and Region

Bin	Country or Territory	Combatant Command	World Bank Geographic Region Classification	Income Group	*N* of Countries in Bin
EAP-1	Cambodia	PACOM	East Asia and Pacific	Low income	2
	Democratic People's Republic of Korea (North Korea)	PACOM	East Asia and Pacific	Low income	
EAP-2	Indonesia	PACOM	East Asia and Pacific	Lower middle income	12
	Kiribati	PACOM	East Asia and Pacific	Lower middle income	
	Laos	PACOM	East Asia and Pacific	Lower middle income	
	Micronesia	PACOM	East Asia and Pacific	Lower middle income	
	Myanmar (Burma)	PACOM	East Asia and Pacific	Lower middle income	
	Papua New Guinea	PACOM	East Asia and Pacific	Lower middle income	
	Philippines	PACOM	East Asia and Pacific	Lower middle income	

Table B.1—Continued

Bin	Country or Territory	Combatant Command	World Bank Geographic Region Classification	Income Group	N of Countries in Bin
	Samoa	PACOM	East Asia and Pacific	Lower middle income	
	Solomon Islands	PACOM	East Asia and Pacific	Lower middle income	
	Timor-Leste (East Timor)	PACOM	East Asia and Pacific	Lower middle income	
	Vanuatu	PACOM	East Asia and Pacific	Lower middle income	
	Vietnam	PACOM	East Asia and Pacific	Lower middle income	
EAP-3	China	PACOM	East Asia and Pacific	Upper middle income	9
	Fiji	PACOM	East Asia and Pacific	Upper middle income	
	Malaysia	PACOM	East Asia and Pacific	Upper middle income	
	Marshall Islands	PACOM	East Asia and Pacific	Upper middle income	
	Mongolia	PACOM	East Asia and Pacific	Upper middle income	
	Palau	PACOM	East Asia and Pacific	Upper middle income	
	Thailand	PACOM	East Asia and Pacific	Upper middle income	
	Tonga	PACOM	East Asia and Pacific	Upper middle income	
	Tuvalu	PACOM	East Asia and Pacific	Upper middle income	
EAP-4	Brunei (Brunei Darussalam)	PACOM	East Asia and Pacific	High income, non-OECD	3
	Singapore	PACOM	East Asia and Pacific	High income, non-OECD	
	Taiwan	PACOM	East Asia and Pacific	High income: non-OECD	
EAP-5	Australia	PACOM	East Asia and Pacific	High income, OECD	4
	Japan	PACOM	East Asia and Pacific	High income, OECD	

Table B.1—Continued

Bin	Country or Territory	Combatant Command	World Bank Geographic Region Classification	Income Group	N of Countries in Bin
	Republic of Korea (South Korea)	PACOM	East Asia and Pacific	High income, OECD	
	New Zealand	PACOM	East Asia and Pacific	High income, OECD	
ECA-1	Armenia	EUCOM	Europe and Central Asia	Lower middle income	8
	Georgia	EUCOM	Europe and Central Asia	Lower middle income	
	Kosovo	EUCOM	Europe and Central Asia	Lower middle income	
	Kyrgyzstan	CENTCOM	Europe and Central Asia	Lower middle income	
	Republic of Moldova	EUCOM	Europe and Central Asia	Lower middle income	
	Tajikistan	CENTCOM	Europe and Central Asia	Lower middle income	
	Ukraine	EUCOM	Europe and Central Asia	Lower middle income	
	Uzbekistan	CENTCOM	Europe and Central Asia	Lower middle income	
ECA-2	Albania	EUCOM	Europe and Central Asia	Upper middle income	12
	Azerbaijan	EUCOM	Europe and Central Asia	Upper middle income	
	Belarus	EUCOM	Europe and Central Asia	Upper middle income	
	Bosnia and Herzegovina	EUCOM	Europe and Central Asia	Upper middle income	
	Bulgaria	EUCOM	Europe and Central Asia	Upper middle income	
	Kazakhstan	CENTCOM	Europe and Central Asia	Upper middle income	
	Macedonia (FYROM)	EUCOM	Europe and Central Asia	Upper middle income	
	Montenegro	EUCOM	Europe and Central Asia	Upper middle income	
	Romania	EUCOM	Europe and Central Asia	Upper middle income	

Table B.1—Continued

Bin	Country or Territory	Combatant Command	World Bank Geographic Region Classification	Income Group	N of Countries in Bin
	Serbia	EUCOM	Europe and Central Asia	Upper middle income	
	Turkey	EUCOM	Europe and Central Asia	Upper middle income	
	Turkmenistan	CENTCOM	Europe and Central Asia	Upper middle income	
ECA-3	Andorra	EUCOM	Europe and Central Asia	High income: non-OECD	9
	Croatia	EUCOM	Europe and Central Asia	High income: non-OECD	
	Cyprus	EUCOM	Europe and Central Asia	High income: non-OECD	
	Latvia	EUCOM	Europe and Central Asia	High income: non-OECD	
	Liechtenstein	EUCOM	Europe and Central Asia	High income: non-OECD	
	Lithuania	EUCOM	Europe and Central Asia	High income: non-OECD	
	Monaco	EUCOM	Europe and Central Asia	High income: non-OECD	
	Russia	EUCOM	Europe and Central Asia	High income: non-OECD	
	San Marino	EUCOM	Europe and Central Asia	High income: non-OECD	
ECA-4	Austria	EUCOM	Europe and Central Asia	High income: OECD	24
	Belgium	EUCOM	Europe and Central Asia	High income: OECD	
	Czech Republic	EUCOM	Europe and Central Asia	High income: OECD	
	Denmark	EUCOM	Europe and Central Asia	High income: OECD	
	Estonia	EUCOM	Europe and Central Asia	High income: OECD	
	Finland	EUCOM	Europe and Central Asia	High income: OECD	
	France	EUCOM	Europe and Central Asia	High income: OECD	

Table B.1—Continued

Bin	Country or Territory	Combatant Command	World Bank Geographic Region Classification	Income Group	N of Countries in Bin
	Germany	EUCOM	Europe and Central Asia	High income: OECD	
	Greece	EUCOM	Europe and Central Asia	High income: OECD	
	Hungary	EUCOM	Europe and Central Asia	High income: OECD	
	Iceland	EUCOM	Europe and Central Asia	High income: OECD	
	Ireland	EUCOM	Europe and Central Asia	High income: OECD	
	Italy	EUCOM	Europe and Central Asia	High income: OECD	
	Luxembourg	EUCOM	Europe and Central Asia	High income: OECD	
	Netherlands	EUCOM	Europe and Central Asia	High income: OECD	
	Norway	EUCOM	Europe and Central Asia	High income: OECD	
	Poland	EUCOM	Europe and Central Asia	High income: OECD	
	Portugal	EUCOM	Europe and Central Asia	High income: OECD	
	Slovakia	EUCOM	Europe and Central Asia	High income: OECD	
	Slovenia	EUCOM	Europe and Central Asia	High income: OECD	
	Spain	EUCOM	Europe and Central Asia	High income: OECD	
	Sweden	EUCOM	Europe and Central Asia	High income: OECD	
	Switzerland	EUCOM	Europe and Central Asia	High income: OECD	
	United Kingdom	EUCOM	Europe and Central Asia	High income: OECD	
LAC-1	Haiti	SOUTHCOM	Latin America and Caribbean	Low income	1
LAC-2	Bolivia	SOUTHCOM	Latin America and Caribbean	Lower middle income	6

Table B.1—Continued

Bin	Country or Territory	Combatant Command	World Bank Geographic Region Classification	Income Group	N of Countries in Bin
	El Salvador	SOUTHCOM	Latin America and Caribbean	Lower middle income	
	Guatemala	SOUTHCOM	Latin America and Caribbean	Lower middle income	
	Guyana	SOUTHCOM	Latin America and Caribbean	Lower middle income	
	Honduras	SOUTHCOM	Latin America and Caribbean	Lower middle income	
	Nicaragua	SOUTHCOM	Latin America and Caribbean	Lower middle income	
LAC-3	Belize	SOUTHCOM	Latin America and Caribbean	Upper middle income	17
	Brazil	SOUTHCOM	Latin America and Caribbean	Upper middle income	
	Colombia	SOUTHCOM	Latin America and Caribbean	Upper middle income	
	Costa Rica	SOUTHCOM	Latin America and Caribbean	Upper middle income	
	Cuba	SOUTHCOM	Latin America and Caribbean	Upper middle income	
	Dominica	SOUTHCOM	Latin America and Caribbean	Upper middle income	
	Dominican Republic	SOUTHCOM	Latin America and Caribbean	Upper middle income	
	Ecuador	SOUTHCOM	Latin America and Caribbean	Upper middle income	
	Grenada	SOUTHCOM	Latin America and Caribbean	Upper middle income	
	Jamaica	SOUTHCOM	Latin America and Caribbean	Upper middle income	
	Mexico	NORTHCOM	Latin America and Caribbean	Upper middle income	
	Panama	SOUTHCOM	Latin America and Caribbean	Upper middle income	
	Paraguay	SOUTHCOM	Latin America and Caribbean	Upper middle income	
	Peru	SOUTHCOM	Latin America and Caribbean	Upper middle income	

Table B.1—Continued

Bin	Country or Territory	Combatant Command	World Bank Geographic Region Classification	Income Group	N of Countries in Bin
	Saint Lucia	SOUTHCOM	Latin America and Caribbean	Upper middle income	
	Saint Vincent and the Grenadines	SOUTHCOM	Latin America and Caribbean	Upper middle income	
	Suriname	SOUTHCOM	Latin America and Caribbean	Upper middle income	
LAC-4	Antigua and Barbuda	SOUTHCOM	Latin America and Caribbean	High income: non-OECD	8
	Argentina	SOUTHCOM	Latin America and Caribbean	High income: non-OECD	
	Bahamas	NORTHCOM	Latin America and Caribbean	High income: non-OECD	
	Barbados	SOUTHCOM	Latin America and Caribbean	High income: non-OECD	
	Saint Kitts and Nevis	SOUTHCOM	Latin America and Caribbean	High income: non-OECD	
	Trinidad and Tobago	SOUTHCOM	Latin America and Caribbean	High income: non-OECD	
	Uruguay	SOUTHCOM	Latin America and Caribbean	High income: non-OECD	
	Venezuela	SOUTHCOM	Latin America and Caribbean	High income: non-OECD	
LAC-5	Chile	SOUTHCOM	Latin America and Caribbean	High income: OECD	1
MENA-1	Djibouti	AFRICOM	Middle East and North Africa	Lower middle income	6
	Egypt	CENTCOM	Middle East and North Africa	Lower middle income	
	Morocco	AFRICOM	Middle East and North Africa	Lower middle income	
	Palestine	CENTCOM	Middle East and North Africa	Lower middle income	
	Syria	CENTCOM	Middle East and North Africa	Lower middle income	
	Yemen	CENTCOM	Middle East and North Africa	Lower middle income	
MENA-2	Algeria	AFRICOM	Middle East and North Africa	Upper middle income	7

Table B.1—Continued

Bin	Country or Territory	Combatant Command	World Bank Geographic Region Classification	Income Group	*N* of Countries in Bin
	Iran	CENTCOM	Middle East and North Africa	Upper middle income	
	Iraq	CENTCOM	Middle East and North Africa	Upper middle income	
	Jordan	CENTCOM	Middle East and North Africa	Upper middle income	
	Lebanon	CENTCOM	Middle East and North Africa	Upper middle income	
	Libya	AFRICOM	Middle East and North Africa	Upper middle income	
	Tunisia	AFRICOM	Middle East and North Africa	Upper middle income	
MENA-3	Bahrain	CENTCOM	Middle East and North Africa	High income: non-OECD	7
	Kuwait	CENTCOM	Middle East and North Africa	High income: non-OECD	
	Malta	EUCOM	Middle East and North Africa	High income: non-OECD	
	Oman	CENTCOM	Middle East and North Africa	High income: non-OECD	
	Qatar	CENTCOM	Middle East and North Africa	High income: non-OECD	
	Saudi Arabia	CENTCOM	Middle East and North Africa	High income: non-OECD	
	United Arab Emirates	CENTCOM	Middle East and North Africa	High income: non-OECD	
MENA-4	Israel	EUCOM	Middle East and North Africa	High income: OECD	1
NA-1	Canada	NORTHCOM	North America	High income: OECD	2
	United States	NORTHCOM	North America	High income: OECD	
SA-1	Afghanistan	CENTCOM	South Asia	Low income	2
	Nepal	PACOM	South Asia	Low income	
SA-2	Bangladesh	PACOM	South Asia	Lower middle income	5
	Bhutan	PACOM	South Asia	Lower middle income	

Table B.1—Continued

Bin	Country or Territory	Combatant Command	World Bank Geographic Region Classification	Income Group	*N* of Countries in Bin
	India	PACOM	South Asia	Lower middle income	
	Pakistan	CENTCOM	South Asia	Lower middle income	
	Sri Lanka	PACOM	South Asia	Lower middle income	
SA-3	Maldives	PACOM	South Asia	Upper middle income	1
SSA-1	Benin	AFRICOM	Sub-Saharan Africa	Low income	26
	Burkina Faso	AFRICOM	Sub-Saharan Africa	Low income	
	Burundi	AFRICOM	Sub-Saharan Africa	Low income	
	Central African Republic	AFRICOM	Sub-Saharan Africa	Low income	
	Chad	AFRICOM	Sub-Saharan Africa	Low income	
	Comoros	AFRICOM	Sub-Saharan Africa	Low income	
	Democratic Republic of the Congo	AFRICOM	Sub-Saharan Africa	Low income	
	Eritrea	AFRICOM	Sub-Saharan Africa	Low income	
	Ethiopia	AFRICOM	Sub-Saharan Africa	Low income	
	The Gambia	AFRICOM	Sub-Saharan Africa	Low income	
	Guinea	AFRICOM	Sub-Saharan Africa	Low income	
	Guinea-Bissau	AFRICOM	Sub-Saharan Africa	Low income	
	Liberia	AFRICOM	Sub-Saharan Africa	Low income	
	Madagascar	AFRICOM	Sub-Saharan Africa	Low income	
	Malawi	AFRICOM	Sub-Saharan Africa	Low income	
	Mali	AFRICOM	Sub-Saharan Africa	Low income	
	Mozambique	AFRICOM	Sub-Saharan Africa	Low income	
	Niger	AFRICOM	Sub-Saharan Africa	Low income	
	Rwanda	AFRICOM	Sub-Saharan Africa	Low income	
	Sierra Leone	AFRICOM	Sub-Saharan Africa	Low income	
	Somalia	AFRICOM	Sub-Saharan Africa	Low income	
	South Sudan	AFRICOM	Sub-Saharan Africa	Low income	

Table B.1—Continued

Bin	Country or Territory	Combatant Command	World Bank Geographic Region Classification	Income Group	N of Countries in Bin
	Tanzania	AFRICOM	Sub-Saharan Africa	Low income	
	Togo	AFRICOM	Sub-Saharan Africa	Low income	
	Uganda	AFRICOM	Sub-Saharan Africa	Low income	
	Zimbabwe	AFRICOM	Sub-Saharan Africa	Low income	
SSA-2	Cameroon	AFRICOM	Sub-Saharan Africa	Lower middle income	14
	Cape Verde	AFRICOM	Sub-Saharan Africa	Lower middle income	
	Republic of the Congo (Congo-Brazzaville)	AFRICOM	Sub-Saharan Africa	Lower middle income	
	Côte d'Ivoire	AFRICOM	Sub-Saharan Africa	Lower middle income	
	Ghana	AFRICOM	Sub-Saharan Africa	Lower middle income	
	Kenya	AFRICOM	Sub-Saharan Africa	Lower middle income	
	Lesotho	AFRICOM	Sub-Saharan Africa	Lower middle income	
	Mauritania	AFRICOM	Sub-Saharan Africa	Lower middle income	
	Nigeria	AFRICOM	Sub-Saharan Africa	Lower middle income	
	São Tomé and Príncipe	AFRICOM	Sub-Saharan Africa	Lower middle income	
	Senegal	AFRICOM	Sub-Saharan Africa	Lower middle income	
	Sudan	AFRICOM	Sub-Saharan Africa	Lower middle income	
	Swaziland	AFRICOM	Sub-Saharan Africa	Lower middle income	
	Zambia	AFRICOM	Sub-Saharan Africa	Lower middle income	
SSA-3	Angola	AFRICOM	Sub-Saharan Africa	Upper middle income	6
	Botswana	AFRICOM	Sub-Saharan Africa	Upper middle income	

Table B.1—Continued

Bin	Country or Territory	Combatant Command	World Bank Geographic Region Classification	Income Group	*N* of Countries in Bin
	Gabon	AFRICOM	Sub-Saharan Africa	Upper middle income	
	Mauritius	AFRICOM	Sub-Saharan Africa	Upper middle income	
	Namibia	AFRICOM	Sub-Saharan Africa	Upper middle income	
	South Africa	AFRICOM	Sub-Saharan Africa	Upper middle income	
SSA-4	Equatorial Guinea	AFRICOM	Sub-Saharan Africa	High income: non-OECD	2
	Seychelles	AFRICOM	Sub-Saharan Africa	High income: non-OECD	

NOTE: Colors in the bin, country or territory, and income group columns reflect the income group; colors in the combatant command and region classification columns reflect the DoD combatant command and World Bank region.

Abbreviations

AFRICOM	U.S. Africa Command
CDC	Centers for Disease Control and Prevention
CENTCOM	U.S. Central Command
DD	disease dynamics
DG	demographic
DoD	U.S. Department of Defense
DRC	Democratic Republic of the Congo
EC	economic
EUCOM	U.S. European Command
GDP	gross domestic product
GHSA	Global Health Security Agenda
HC	health care
HHS	U.S. Department of Health and Human Services
IHR	International Health Regulations
NGO	nongovernmental organization
NORTHCOM	U.S. Northern Command
OECD	Organisation for Economic Co-operation and Development
PACOM	U.S. Pacific Command
P-D	political-domestic

PH   public health

P-I   political-international

SOUTHCOM   U.S. Southern Command

USAID   U.S. Agency for International Development

WHO   World Health Organization

Data Sources

Demographic

United Nations, *World Urbanization Prospects*, 2014. As of February 21, 2016:
http://esa.un.org/unpd/wup/DataQuery/

World Bank, "Adult Literacy Rate, Population 15+ Years, Both Sexes (%)," 2013. As of February 21, 2016:
http://data.worldbank.org/indicator/SE.ADT.LITR.ZS

World Bank, "Literacy Rate, Adult Female, (% of Females Ages 15 and Above)," 2013. As of February 21, 2016:
http://data.worldbank.org/indicator/SE.ADT.LITR.FE.ZS

World Bank, "Net Migration," 2012. As of February 21, 2016:
http://data.worldbank.org/indicator/SM.POP.NETM?display=default

World Bank, "Population Density (People per Sq. km of Land Area)," 2014. As of February 21, 2016:
http://data.worldbank.org/indicator/EN.POP.DNST

World Bank, "Population Growth (Annual %)," 2014. As of February 21, 2016:
http://data.worldbank.org/indicator/SP.POP.GROW?display=default

Health Care

World Bank, "Health Expenditure, Total (% of GDP)," 2013. As of February 21, 2016:
http://data.worldbank.org/indicator/SH.XPD.TOTL.ZS/countries/1W?display=default

World Bank, "Health Expenditure Per Capita (Current US$)," 2013. As of February 21, 2016:
http://data.worldbank.org/indicator/SH.XPD.PCAP/countries/1W?display=default

World Health Organization, "Density of Nursing and Midwifery Personnel (Total Number per 1000 Population, Latest Available Year)," most recent year available considering 1998–2014. As of February 21, 2016:
http://www.who.int/gho/health_workforce/nursing_midwifery_density/en/

World Health Organization, "Density of Physicians (Total Number per 1000 Population, Latest Available Year)," most recent year available considering 1998–2014. As of February 21, 2016:
http://www.who.int/gho/health_workforce/physicians_density/en/

World Health Organization, "Health Infrastructure: Data by Country," health centers per 100,000 population, 2013. As of February 21, 2016:
http://apps.who.int/gho/data/node.main.506?lang=en

World Health Organization, "Health Infrastructure: Data by Country," hospital beds per 1,000 population, 2011. As of February 21, 2016:
http://apps.who.int/gho/data/node.main.506?lang=en

World Health Organization, "Number of Deaths (Thousands): Data by Country," infant mortality rate (number of deaths in <12 months per 1,000 livebirths), 2015. As of February 21, 2016:
http://apps.who.int/gho/data/view.main.CM1320N?lang=en

Public Health

Centers for Disease Control and Prevention, "Global Health—CDC and the Global Health Security Agenda," 2016. As of February 21, 2016:
http://www.cdc.gov/globalhealth/security/index.htm

International Association of National Public Health Institutes, "Our Members," 2016. As of February 21, 2016:
http://www.ianphi.org/membercountries/index.html

World Health Organization, "Diphtheria Tetanus Toxoid and Pertussis (DTP3): Data by Country," 2014. As of February 21, 2016:
http://apps.who.int/gho/data/node.main.A827

World Health Organization, "International Health Regulations (2005) Monitoring Framework," 2014 data. As of February 21, 2016:
http://www.who.int/gho/ihr/en/

World Health Organization, "Measles (MCV): Data by Country," 2014. As of February 21, 2016:
http://apps.who.int/gho/data/view.main.80100

World Health Organization, "Population Using Improved Drinking Water Sources (%)," 2012. As of February 21, 2016:
http://apps.who.int/gho/data/node.main.46?lang=en

World Health Organization, "Population Using Improved Sanitation Facilities (%)." As of February 21, 2016:
http://apps.who.int/gho/data/node.main.46?lang=en

Disease Dynamics

World Bank, "Agricultural Land (% of Land Area)," 2012. As of February 21, 2016:
http://data.worldbank.org/indicator/AG.LND.AGRI.ZS/countries

World Bank, "Average Precipitation in Depth (mm per Year)," 2014. As of February 21, 2016:
http://data.worldbank.org/indicator/AG.LND.PRCP.MM

World Bank, "Climate Change Knowledge Portal: Historical Data," annual average temperature, 1961–1999. As of February 21, 2016:
http://data.worldbank.org/data-catalog/cckp_historical_data

World Bank, "Forest Area (% of Land Area)," 2012. As of February 21, 2016:
http://data.worldbank.org/indicator/AG.LND.FRST.ZS

Political-Domestic

Amnesty International, The Political Terror Scale. As of December 3, 2015:
http://www.politicalterrorscale.org/

Fund for Peace, Fragile States Index, 2013. As of July 25, 2016:
http://fsi.fundforpeace.org/rankings-2013-sortable

Ivanyna, Maksym, and Anwar Shah, "How Close Is Your Government to Its People? Worldwide Indicators on Localization and Decentralization," July 1, 2012, World Bank Policy Research Working Paper No. 6138. As of December 3, 2015:
http://papers.ssrn.com/sol3/papers.cfm?abstract_id=2112806

Polity IV Project: Political Regime Characteristics and Transitions, 1800–2013, 2014. As of December 3, 2015:
http://www.systemicpeace.org/polity/polity4.htm

Transparency International, Corruption Perceptions Index, 2014. As of December 3, 2015:
http://www.transparency.org/cpi2014

United Nations Development Programme, "Human Development Data, 1980–2015." As of December 2, 2015:
http://hdr.undp.org/en/data

World Bank, Worldwide Governance Indicators. As of December 2, 2015:
http://info.worldbank.org/governance/wgi/index.aspx#home

Political-International

Global Health Data Exchange, Development Assistance for Health Database 1990–2011. As of December 7, 2015:
http://ghdx.healthdata.org/record/development-assistance-health-database-1990-2011

IHS, Jane's Country Risk Intelligence Centre Module. As of December 7, 2015:
http://www.janes.com/

United Nations Development Programme, "Our Projects." As of December 7, 2015:
http://open.undp.org/#2015

World Bank, "Net Official Development Assistance and Official Aid Received (Current US$)," 1960–2014. As of December 7, 2015:
http://data.worldbank.org/indicator/DT.ODA.ALLD.CD

World Bank, "Net ODA Received (% GNI)," 1960–2014 As of December 7, 2015:
http://data.worldbank.org/indicator/DT.ODA.ODAT.GN.ZS

Economic

Humanitarian Data Exchange, "Poverty Headcount Ratio at $1.25 a Day (PPP)." As of December 2, 2015:
https://data.hdx.rwlabs.org/dataset/poverty_headcount_ratio_at_125_a_day_ppp

Nation Master, "Media > Televisions per 1000: Countries Compared," 2003. As of December 2, 2015:
http://www.nationmaster.com/country-info/stats/Media/Televisions-per-1000

Nation Master, "Transport > Roads > Paved > % of Total Roads: Countries Compared," percentage of total roads paved. As of December 2, 2015:
http://www.nationmaster.com/country-info/stats/Transport/Roads/Paved/%25-of-total-roads

World Bank, "Foreign Direct Investment, Net Inflows (BoP, Current US$)," 1970–2015. As of December 2, 2015:
http://data.worldbank.org/indicator/BX.KLT.DINV.CD.WD/countries

World Bank, "GDP Per Capita (Current US$)," 1960–2015. As of December 2, 2015:
http://data.worldbank.org/indicator/NY.GDP.PCAP.CD

World Bank, "GDP Per Capita Growth (Annual %)," 1961–2015. As of December 2, 2015:
http://data.worldbank.org/indicator/NY.GDP.PCAP.KD.ZG

World Bank, "Internet Users (per 100 People)," 1990–2014. As of December 2, 2015:
http://data.worldbank.org/indicator/IT.NET.USER.P2/countries

World Bank, "Knowledge Economy Index," 2012. As of December 2, 2015:
http://data.worldbank.org/data-catalog/KEI

World Bank, "Mobile Cellular Subscriptions (per 100 People)," 1960–2014. As of December 2, 2015:
http://data.worldbank.org/indicator/IT.CEL.SETS.P2

Bibliography

Miscellaneous Works Cited in Text

CDC—*See* Centers for Disease Control and Prevention.

Centers for Disease Control and Prevention, "2014 Ebola Outbreak in West Africa—Case Counts," web page, updated April 23, 2016. As of July 11, 2016:
https://www.cdc.gov/vhf/ebola/outbreaks/2014-west-africa/case-counts.html

Chamberlin, Margaret, Adeyemi Okunogbe, Melinda Moore, and Mahshid Abir, *Intra-Action Report—A Dynamic Tool for Emergency Managers and Policymakers: A Proof of Concept and Illustrative Application to the 2014–2015 Ebola Crisis*, Santa Monica, Calif.: RAND Corporation, PE-147-RC, 2015. As of July 1, 2016:
http://www.rand.org/pubs/perspectives/PE147.html

Christian, Kira A., Kashef Ijaz, Scott F. Dowell, Catherine C. Chow, Rohit A. Chitale, Joseph S. Bresee, Eric Mintz, Mark A. Pallansch, Steven Wassilak, Eugene McCray, and Ray R. Arthur, "What We Are Watching—Five Top Global Infectious Disease Threats, 2012: A Perspective from CDC's Global Disease Detection Operations Center," *Emerging Health Threats Journal*, Vol. 6, No. 20632, 2013. As of June 14, 2016:
http://dx.doi.org/10.3402/ehtj.v6i0.20632

Gelfeld, Bill, Shira Efron, Melinda Moore, and Jonah Blank, *Mitigating the Impact of Ebola in Potential Hot Zones: A Proof-of-Concept Approach to Help Decisionmakers Prepare for High-Risk Scenarios Outside Guinea, Liberia, and Sierra Leone*, Santa Monica, Calif.: RAND Corporation, PE-146-RC, 2015. As of July 1, 2016:
http://www.rand.org/pubs/perspectives/PE146.html

Hamblin, James, "This Is Resilience," *The Atlantic*, April 4, 2014. As of June 30, 2016:
http://www.theatlantic.com/health/archive/2014/04/this-is-resilience/360181/

HHS—See U.S. Department of Health and Human Services.

Noah, Don, and George Fidas, *Global Infectious Disease Threat and Its Implications for the United States*, Washington, D.C.: National Intelligence Council, 2000. As of June 14, 2016:
http://fas.org/irp/threat/nie99-17d.htm

U.S. Department of Health and Human Services, *National Health Security Strategy and Implementation Plan 2015–2018*, Washington, D.C., 2015. As of June 14, 2016:
http://www.phe.gov/Preparedness/planning/authority/nhss/Documents/nhss-ip.pdf

White House, *Global Health Security: Vision and Overarching Target*, Washington, D.C., 2014. As of December 2, 2015:
http://www.cdc.gov/globalhealth/security/pdf/ghs_overarching_target.pdf

————, *National Security Strategy*, Washington, D.C., 2015. As of December 2, 2015:
https://www.whitehouse.gov/sites/default/files/docs/2015_national_security_strategy.pdf

WHO—*See* World Health Organization.

World Health Organization, *International Health Regulations*, 2nd ed., Geneva, 2005. As of June 14, 2016:
http://whqlibdoc.who.int/publications/2008/9789241580410_eng.pdf

————, "Statement on the 1st Meeting of the IHR Emergency Committee on the 2014 Ebola Outbreak in West Africa," August 8, 2014a. As of July 25, 2016:
http://www.who.int/mediacentre/news/statements/2014/ebola-20140808/en/

————, "Democratic Republic of the Congo: The Country That Knows How to Beat Ebola," December 2014b. As of July 25, 2016:
http://www.who.int/features/2014/drc-beats-ebola/en/

————, "Lassa Fever—Nigeria," January 27, 2016. As of July 25, 2016:
http://who.int/csr/don/27-january-2016-lassa-fever-nigeria/en/

Sources by Domain

The following sections, organized by domain, list the sources that were the foundation of the factors and justification for the hypotheses in the report. See Chapter Three.

Demographic

Choffnes, Eileen R., and Alison Mack, *The Influence of Global Environmental Change on Infectious Disease Dynamics: Workshop Summary*, Washington, D.C.: National Academies Press, 2014.

Goenka, Aditya, and Lin Liu, "Infectious Diseases, Human Capital and Economic Growth," mimeo, National University of Singapore and University of Rochester, 2013.

Jones, Kate E., Nikkita G. Patel, Marc A. Levy, Adam Storeygard, Deborah Balk, John L. Gittleman, and Peter Daszak, "Global Trends in Emerging Infectious Diseases," *Nature*, Vol. 451, No. 7181, 2008, pp. 990–993.

Lederberg, Joshua, Margaret A. Hamburg, and Mark S. Smolinski, *Microbial Threats to Health: Emergence, Detection, and Response*, Washington, D.C.: National Academies Press, 2003.

Health Care

Clements, Archie, Kate Halton, Nicholas Graves, Anthony Pettitt, Anthony Morton, David Looke, and Michael Whitby, "Overcrowding and Understaffing in Modern Health-Care Systems: Key Determinants in Meticillin-Resistant Staphylococcus Aureus Transmission," *The Lancet Infectious Diseases*, Vol. 8, No. 7, 2008, pp. 427–434.

Coker, Richard J., Benjamin M. Hunter, James W. Rudge, Marco Liverani, and Piya Hanvoravongchai, "Emerging Infectious Diseases in Southeast Asia: Regional Challenges to Control," *The Lancet*, Vol. 377, No. 9765, 2011, pp. 599–609.

Noah, Don, and George Fidas, *The Global Infectious Disease Threat and Its Implications for the United States*, Washington, D.C.: National Intelligence Council, 2000. As of June 14, 2016:
http://fas.org/irp/threat/nie99-17d.htm

Public Health

Berkelman, Ruth L., Ralph T. Bryan, Michael T. Osterholm, James W. LeDuc, and Jim M. Hughes, "Infectious Disease Surveillance: A Crumbling Foundation," *Science*, Vol. 264, No. 5157, 1994, pp. 368–370.

Centers for Disease Control and Prevention, "Global Health—CDC and the Global Health Security Agenda," web page, last updated February 11, 2016. As of February 21, 2016: http://www.cdc.gov/globalhealth/security/index.htm

Coker, Richard J., Benjamin M. Hunter, James W. Rudge, Marco Liverani, and Piya Hanvoravongchai, "Emerging Infectious Diseases in Southeast Asia: Regional Challenges to Control," *The Lancet*, Vol. 377, No. 9765, 2011, pp. 599–609.

Gostin, L. O., S. Burris, and Z. Lazzarini, "The Law and the Public's Health: A Study of Infectious Disease Law in the United States," *Columbia Law Review*, Vol. 99, No. 1, 1999, pp. 59–128.

Lederberg, Joshua, Margaret A. Hamburg, and Mark S. Smolinski, *Microbial Threats to Health: Emergence, Detection, and Response*, Washington, D.C.: National Academies Press, 2003.

Morse, Stephen S., "Factors in the Emergence of Infectious Diseases," in Andrew T. Price-Smith, ed., *Plagues and Politics: Infectious Disease and International Policy*, New York: Palgrave, 2001.

Smith, Richard D., "Responding to Global Infectious Disease Outbreaks: Lessons from SARS on the Role of Risk Perception, Communication and Management," *Social Science and Medicine*, Vol. 63, No. 12, 2006, pp. 3113–3123.

United Nations, "World Population Prospects, the 2015 Revision," web page, 2015. As of July 7, 2016: https://esa.un.org/unpd/wpp/

Disease Dynamics

Choffnes, Eileen R., and Alison Mack, *The Influence of Global Environmental Change on Infectious Disease Dynamics: Workshop Summary*, Washington, D.C.: National Academies Press, 2014.

Geller, Laurie, "Under the Weather: Climate, Ecosystems, and Infectious Disease," *Emerging Infectious Diseases*, Vol. 7, No. 7, June 2001. As of July 7, 2016: http://wwwnc.cdc.gov/eid/article/7/7/01-7750_article

Jones, Kate E., Nikkita G. Patel, Marc A. Levy, Adam Storeygard, Deborah Balk, John L. Gittleman, and Peter Daszak, "Global Trends in Emerging Infectious Diseases," *Nature*, Vol. 451, No. 7181, 2008, pp. 990–993.

Kilpatrick, A. Marm, and Sarah E. Randolph, "Drivers, Dynamics, and Control of Emerging Vector-Borne Zoonotic Diseases," *The Lancet*, Vol. 380, No. 9857, 2012, pp. 1946–1955.

Morse, Stephen S., "Factors in the Emergence of Infectious Diseases," in Andrew T. Price-Smith, ed., *Plagues and Politics: Infectious Disease and International Policy*, New York: Palgrave, 2001.

Morse, Stephen S., Jonna A. K. Mazet, Mark Woolhouse, Colin R. Parrish, Dennis Carroll, William B. Karesh, Carlos Zambrana-Torrelio, W. Ian Lipkinand, and Peter Daszak, "Prediction and Prevention of the Next Pandemic Zoonosis," *The Lancet*, Vol. 380, No. 9857, 2012, pp. 1956–1965.

Patz, Jonathan A., Peter Daszak, Gary M. Tabor, A. Alonso Aguirre, Mary Pearl, Jon Epstein, Nathan D. Wolfe, A. Marm Kilpatrick, Johannes Foufopoulos, David Molyneux, and David J. Bradley, "Unhealthy Lndscapes: Policy Recommendations on Land Use Change and Infectious Disease Emergence," *Environmental Health Perspectives*, Vol. 112, No. 10, 2004, pp. 1092–1098.

Woolhouse, Mark E. J., and Sonya Gowtage-Sequeria, "Host Range and Emerging and Reemerging Pathogens," paper presented at the *Ending the War Metaphor: The Changing Agenda for Unraveling the Host-Microbe Relationship Workshop*, 2006.

Political-Domestic

Besley, Timothy, and Masayuki Kudamatsu, "Health and Democracy," *The American Economic Review*, Vol. 96, No. 2, 2006, pp. 313–318.

Bornemisza, Olga, M. Kent Ranson, Timothy M. Poletti, and Egbert Sondorp, "Promoting Health Equity in Conflict-Affected Fragile States," *Social Science and Medicine*, Vol. 70, No. 1, 2010, pp. 80–88.

Dreze, Jean, and Amartya Kumar Sen, *India: Development and Participation*, New York: Oxford University Press, 2002.

Logie, Dorothy E., Michael Rowson, and Felix Ndagije, "Innovations in Rwanda's Health System: Looking to the Future," *The Lancet*, Vol. 372, No. 9634, 2008, pp. 256–261.

Mann, Johnathan, "Health and Human Rights," *American Journal of Public Health*, November 2006, Vol. 96, No. 11, 2011, pp. 1940–1943.

Mullany, Luke C., Adam K. Richards, Catherine I. Lee, Voravit Suwanvanichkij, Cynthia Maung, Mahn Mahn, Chris Beyrer, and Thomas J. Lee, "Population-Based Survey Methods to Quantify Associations Between Human Rights Violations and Health Outcomes Among Internally Displaced Persons in Eastern Burma," *Journal of Epidemiology and Community Health*, Vol. 61, No. 10, 2007, pp. 908–914.

Phillips, Carleton J., Anne M. Harrington, Terry L. Yates, Gary L. Simpson, and Robert J. Baker, *Global Disease Surveillance, Emergent Disease Preparedness, and National Security*, Lubbock: Museum of Texas Tech University, 2009.

Rajkumar, Andrew Sunil, and Vinaya Swaroop, "Public Spending and Outcomes: Does Governance Matter?" *Journal of Development Economics*, Vol. 86, No. 1, 2008, pp. 96–111.

Robalino, David A., Oscar F. Picazo, and Albertus Voetberg, "Does Fiscal Decentralization Improve Health Outcomes?" working paper, World Bank, March 2001.

Political-International

Hanvoravongchai, Piya, Wiku Adisasmito, Pham N. Chau, Alexandra Conseil, Joia de Sa, Ralf Krumkamp, Sandra Mounier-Jack et al., "Pandemic Influenza Preparedness and Health Systems Challenges in Asia: Results from Rapid Analyses in 6 Asian Countries," *BMC Public Health*, Vol. 10, No. 322, 2010.

Jamison, Dean T., Joel G. Breman, Anthony R. Measham, George Alleyne, Mariam Claeson, David B. Evans, Prabhat Jha, Anne Mills, and Philip Musgrove, eds., *Disease Control Priorities in Developing Countries*, 2nd ed., New York: Oxford University Press; Washington, D.C.: World Bank, 2006.

Mauch, Verena, Diana Weil, Aayid Munim, Francois Boillot, Rudi Coninx, Sevil Huseynova, Clydette Powell, Akihiro Seita, Henriette Wembanyama, and Susan van den Hof, "Structure and Management of Tuberculosis Control Programs in Fragile States—Afghanistan, DR Congo, Haiti, Somalia," *Health Policy*, Vol. 96, No. 2, 2010, pp. 118–127.

McDougall, Christopher W., Ross E. G. Upshur, and Kumanan Wilson, "Emerging Norms for the Control of Emerging Epidemics," *Bulletin of the World Health Organization*, Vol. 86, No. 8, 2008, pp. 643–645.

Economic

Doebbeling, Bradley N., Ann F. Chou, and William M. Tierney, "Priorities and Strategies for the Implementation of Integrated Informatics and Communications Technology to Improve Evidence-Based Practice," *Journal of General Internal Medicine*, Vol. 21, No. S2, 2006, pp. S50–S57.

Goenka, Aditya, and Lin Liu, "Infectious Diseases, Human Capital and Economic Growth," mimeo, National University of Singapore and University of Rochester, 2013.

Levine, Adam C., David Z. Presser, Stephanie Rosborough, Tedros A. Ghebreyesus, and Mark A. Davis, "Understanding Barriers to Emergency Care in Low-Income Countries: View from the Front Line," *Prehospital and Disaster Medicine*, Vol. 22, No. 5, 2007, pp. 467–470.

Pritchett, Lant, and Lawrence H. Summers, "Wealthier Is Healthier," *Journal of Human Resources*, Vol. 31, No. 4, 1996, pp. 841–868.